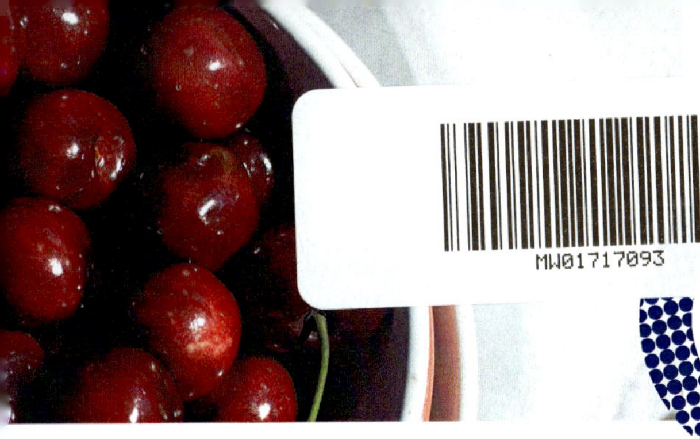

Contents

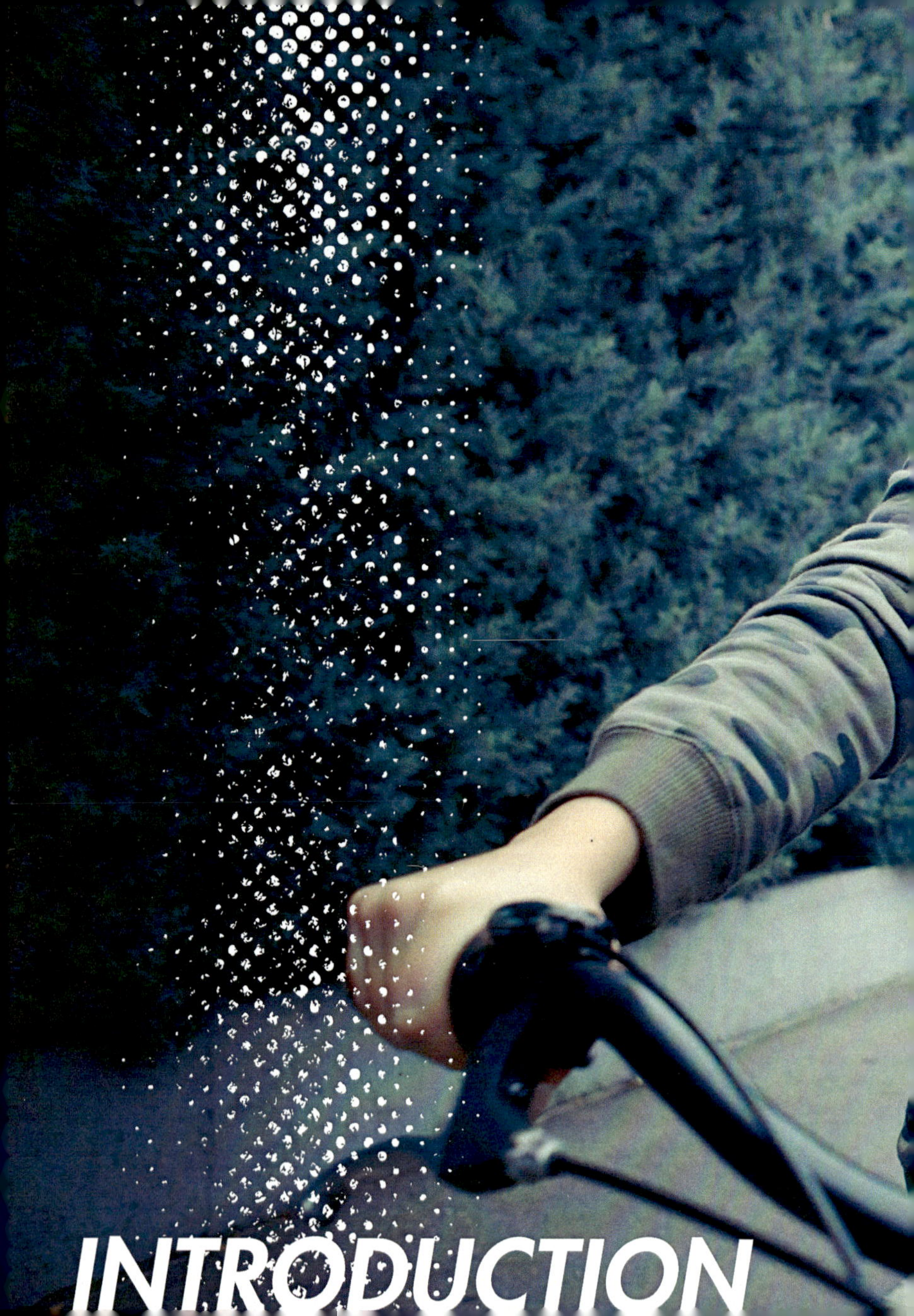

INTRODUCTION

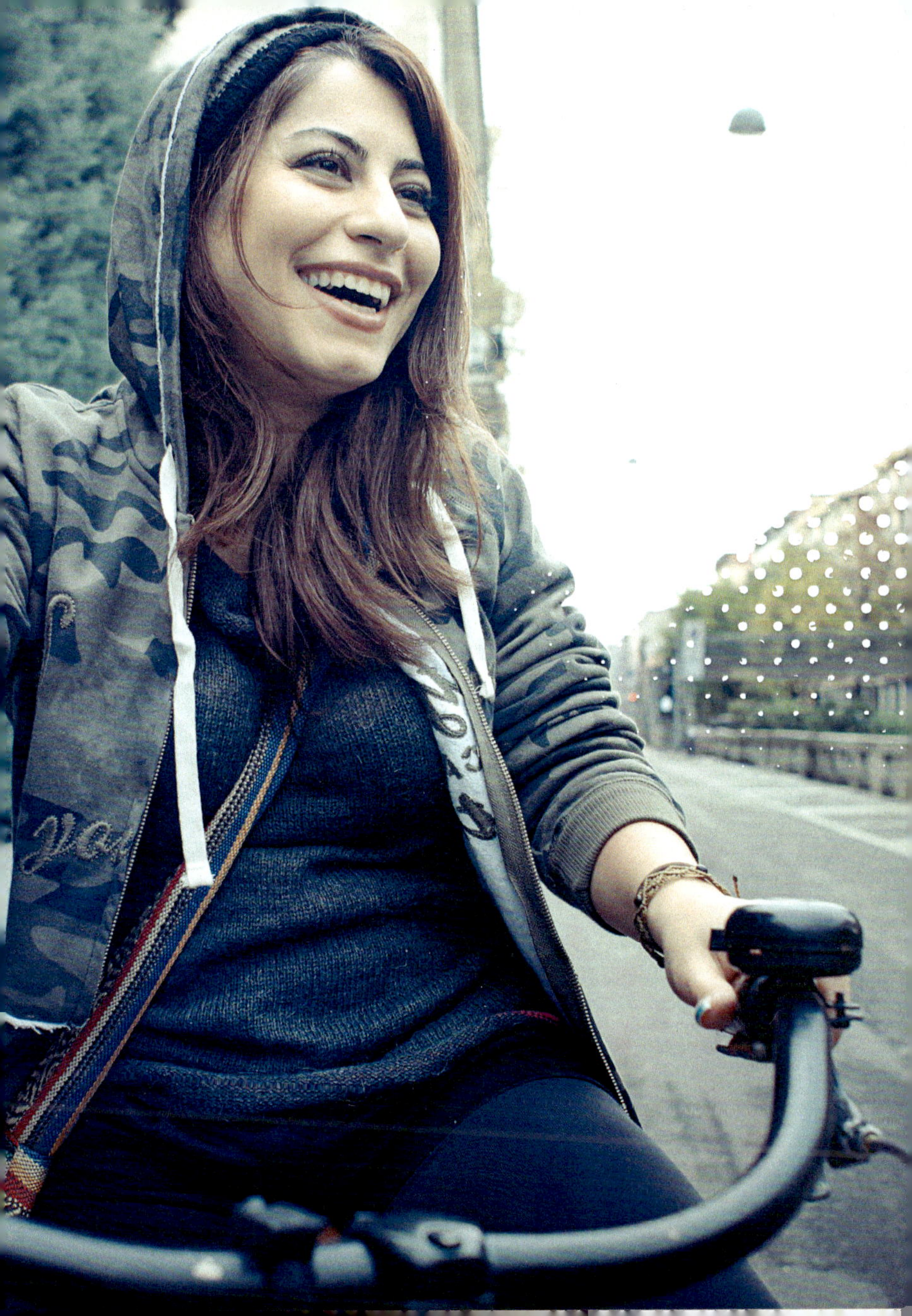

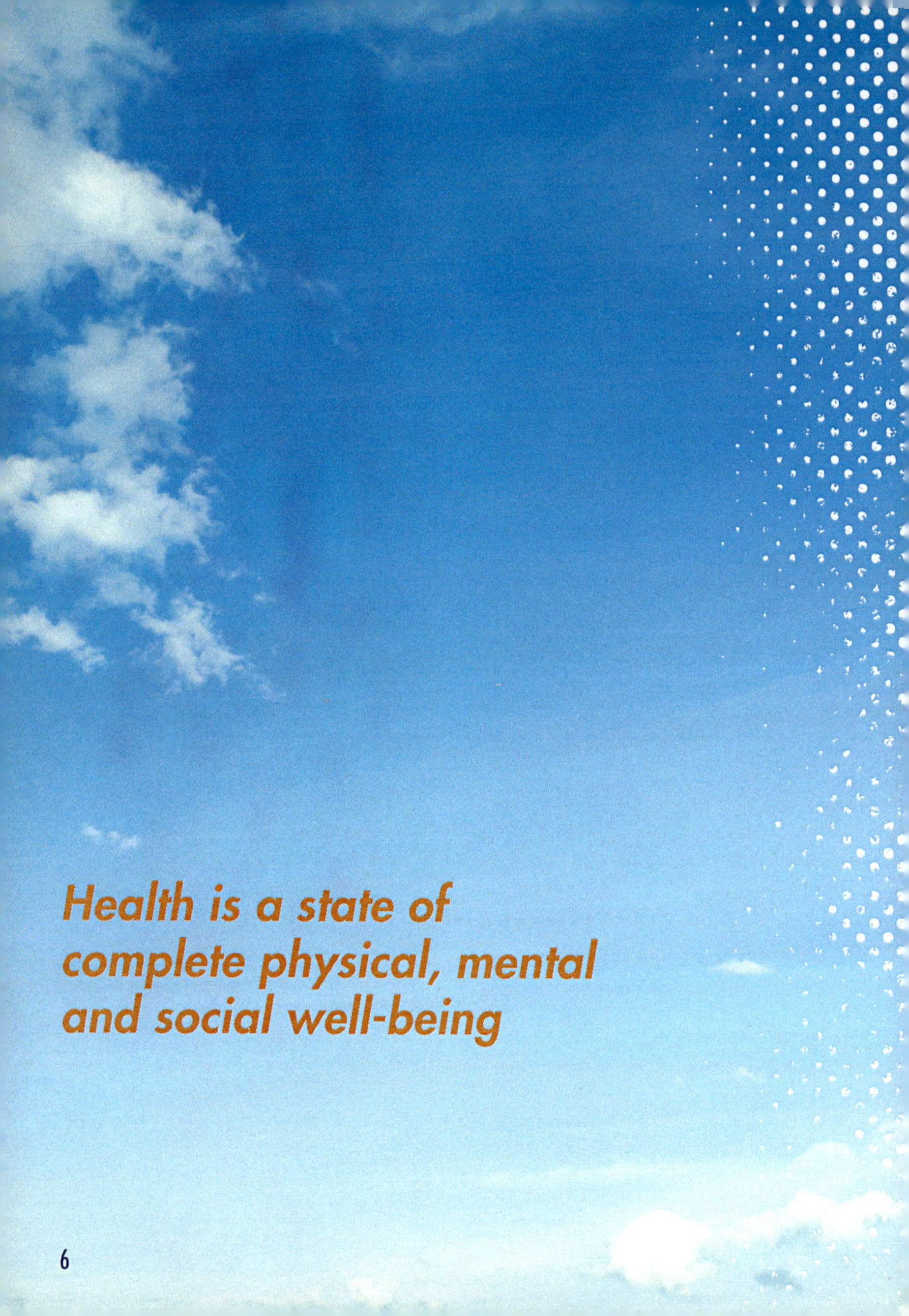

Health is a state of complete physical, mental and social well-being

WHY IT'S TIME FOR A CHANGE

And not just a short term solution.

You're tired of wasting your time, energy and, likely, your money on a quick-fix diet plan, pill or piece of workout equipment promising to change your life - only to find yourself failing again, and back where you started.

And you're not the only one. We see so many health crisis headlines these days we're becoming almost numb to it. But the fact is, we're dying from both obesity and malnutrition. Yes, you read correctly: both.

› *Americans are gaining weight as fast as they are losing health.*

In 1980 an estimated 15% of Americans were obese. Today the Center for Disease Control (CDC) estimates obesity to be at 34.9% and it's expected to increase to 42% by 2030.[1]

› *Why should we care?*

According to the CDC, obesity is associated with heart disease, stroke, Type 2 diabetes, some types of cancer, and continues to be one of America's leading causes of preventable death.[2]

› *We commonly associate being skinny as healthy, but this isn't the full truth.*

Starving yourself into the skinny category causes emotional stress and nutritional deficiencies. Keep in mind thin people can still get cancer and heart disease.

This brings me to the real point of this workbook, and to why it stands out from the other plans you may have followed: Health is a state of complete physical, mental and social well-being. It's not merely the absence of disease or infirmity, nor is it a 'perfect' number on a scale.

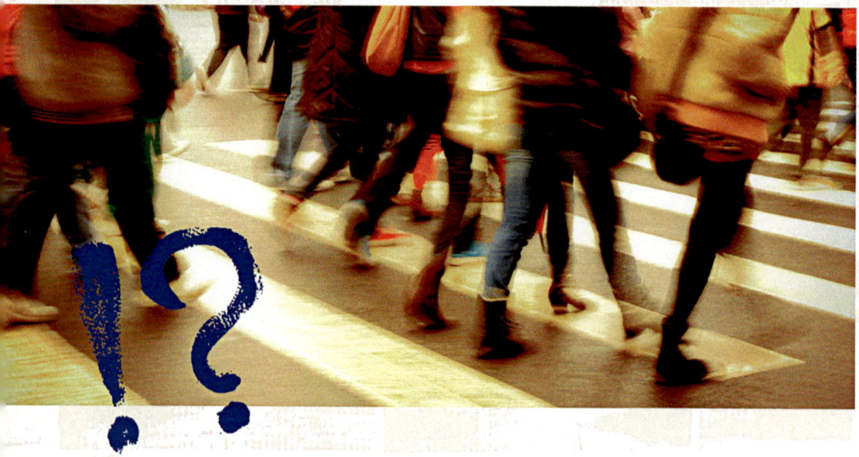

Think on this: Have you ever been in a public place with someone coughing next to you, but you didn't catch their cold? There's no doubt you came in contact with their bacteria or virus. Yet, your body had the ability to overcome the outside threat and remain healthy. It's important to realize diseases and illnesses are not usually caused by one specific thing.

Many cancers are asymptomatic, which is why it's important to do early detection screenings. And, according to the American Heart Association, for 50% of men and 64% of women, the heart attack comes before they learn they have heart disease.[3]

Most disease is multifactorial, coming on because of a combination of genetics, nutritional deficiencies, toxicities, lack of exercise, and high levels of stress over prolonged periods of time. All of these stressors can lower the immune system's ability to adapt and leave the body more susceptible to bacteria, viruses and other types of illness.

Americans like to point a finger at genetics by blaming mom and dad for their high blood pressure, bad cholesterol and sickness. But what if your lifestyle has more influence on your health than genetics?

New research suggests many of our diseases have more to do with lifestyle choices than the family tree. Studies with identical twins have shown different lifestyle choices create different outcomes; one identical twin could get breast cancer while the other twin does not.[5]

According to the American Cancer Society, only 5 to 10 percent of cancers are a direct result of gene defects, which is the type of cancer inherited from your parents. [4]

In other words, if you eat poorly, smoke, or choose other toxic and deficient lifestyle activities, you can trigger your genetics to express disease just as you can trigger healthy genetic expression by living a wellness lifestyle. This is shown in the field of epigenetics, which studies how the environment and lifestyle choices influence genetic expression.

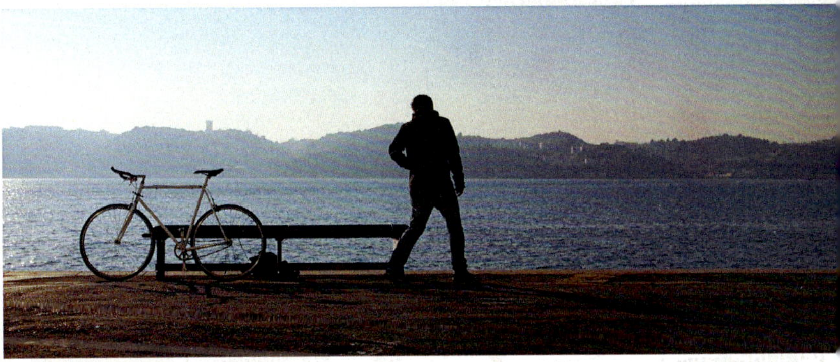

SAY HELLO TO YOUR NEW FRIEND

If you want to be healthy, you need short term results that become a long-term solution. You need a doable and repeatable health program – one to help you create healthy habits.
Anything else is, literally, a waste of time.

Why believe me?

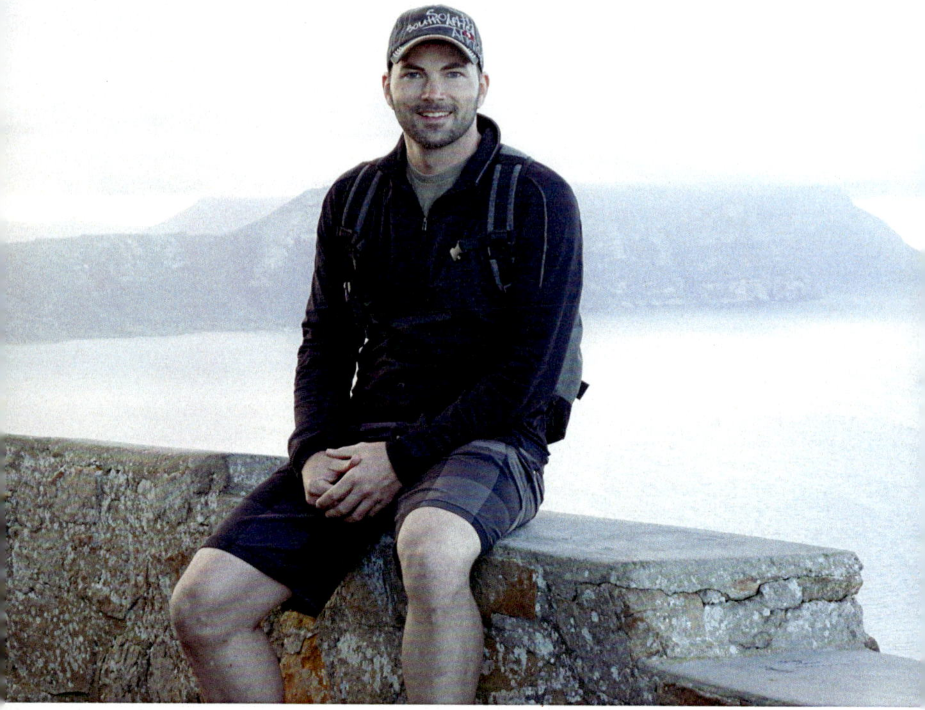

Healthy lifestyle, healthy you

In January of 1999, I was seriously injured physically and emotionally in an automobile collision. This crash caused multiple contusions and fractures, and killed two of my friends. A broken back and fractured leg forced me to walk with crutches followed by several months using a cane. This tragic part of my life will forever be an influence on who I am and what I stand for.

My road to recovery was slow and grueling, but it helped me understand the power of forgiveness, the gift of gratitude, and how heavy the world can be when you hold onto anger, frustration and shame. These are not lessons we can learn overnight. The road from today to tomorrow is never as straight as we would like. Remember to celebrate your successes and handle your setbacks gracefully.

My wellness journey started with accepting I was not invincible. It sent me on a quest for knowledge and eventually led me to Chiropractic College, where I was introduced to Dr. James Chestnut and the Wellness Certification I hold through Life West & the International Chiropractic Association. His certification's foundation along with action has allowed me to remodel my own body-mind and help my patients and community on their own wellness journey. Without his influence the First21 would look like other programs on the market – an all or nothing challenge leading to overwhelmedness and defeat more often than habit forming success.

The First21 was created to be your first steps on a lifetime journey of health and wellness. Based on the principle it takes 21 days to make or break a habit, the First21 works by making things simple. It splits the complexity of wellness into doable health challenges to be carried out over habit-forming periods of time. These challenges are meant to be repeated to help you continually improve, maintain or even to get you back on track.

The First21 is your friend. It's your simple, healthy, achievable new habit.
And it's just within your reach!

Geoff Huls, DC, CCWP

1
THE FIRST21 FOUNDATIONAL CONCEPTS

WHY 21 DAYS?

We are creatures of habit, which means when we like something we want to do it over and over and over again. Sadly, those habits aren't always healthy ones. Take pizza; a favorite food for many Americans. Most of us don't have it occasionally, we have it habitually.

In fact, 93% of Americans have eaten a pizza within the last month, and 16% of men and 13% of women eat pizza daily, according to the USDA [6]

Many people eat the same thing each week and repeat it every week. Imagine how you could benefit from exchanging this habitual act with a healthy one?

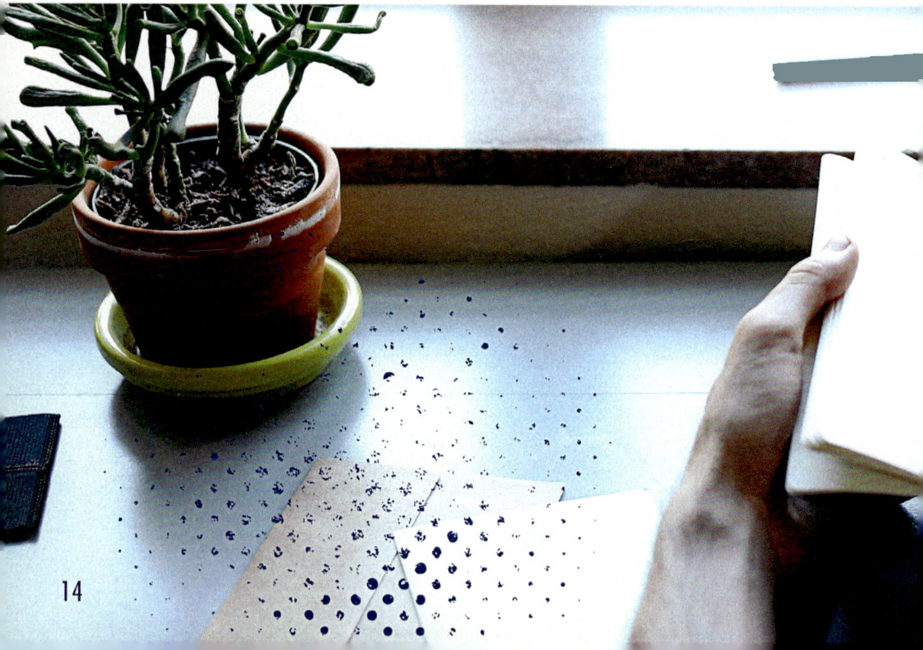

The First21 goes on exactly the same principle. It's just the habits you'll be forming are good for you – for your body, mind and spirit. These challenges were created to be done over 21 days– giving you the opportunity to develop healthy habits without the stress of a long term commitment.

"We are what we repeatedly do. Excellence, therefore, is not an action but a habit." – Aristotle

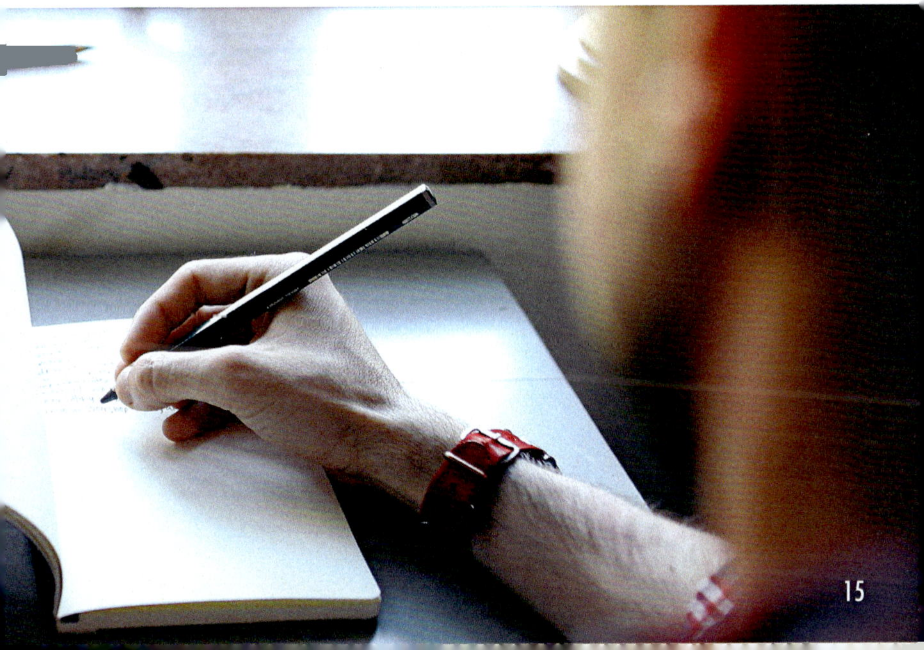

MORE THAN COMMON SENSE

We all know broccoli is better for the body than a candy bar, walking is better than sitting and gratitude is better than anger.

But we also know eating a candy bar is faster than preparing broccoli, sitting is way easier than walking and sometimes we want to like our boss as much as we want to eat broccoli or have time for a walk.

When it comes to health, people do not lack common sense, they lack the action steps and accountability needed to stay or get healthy.

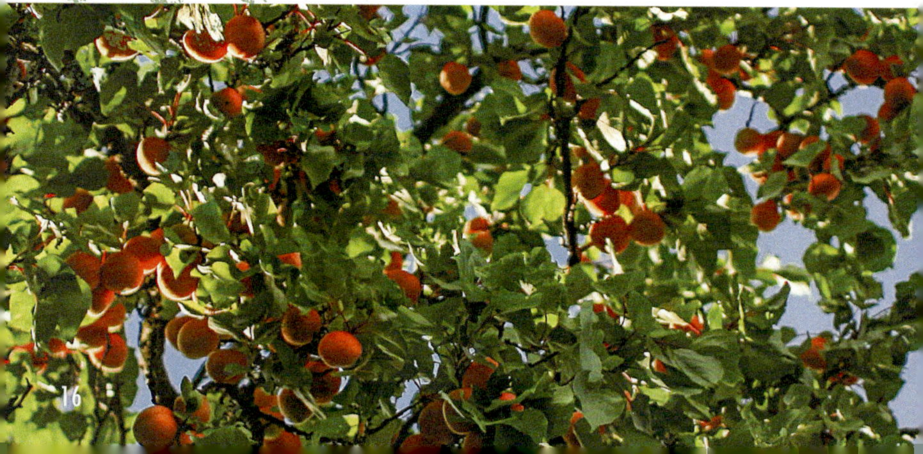

Keeping a diary or journal has been widely proven to be beneficial for your mental and physical health. It's therapeutic, it's a creative outlet, and when it comes to your diet it keeps you accountable.

WHEN SHOULD YOU START?

If you knew you would live to be 90, when would you start living healthfully? This is a question many people should start asking at a younger age, because the body of tomorrow is created today.

It feels good to feel good. This is true even if you are suffering with a chronic condition, because feeling better than you do is better than feeling the same or worse. For this reason alone, it's never too late to make healthy lifestyle changes. It will never be easier for you to take your first steps than now!

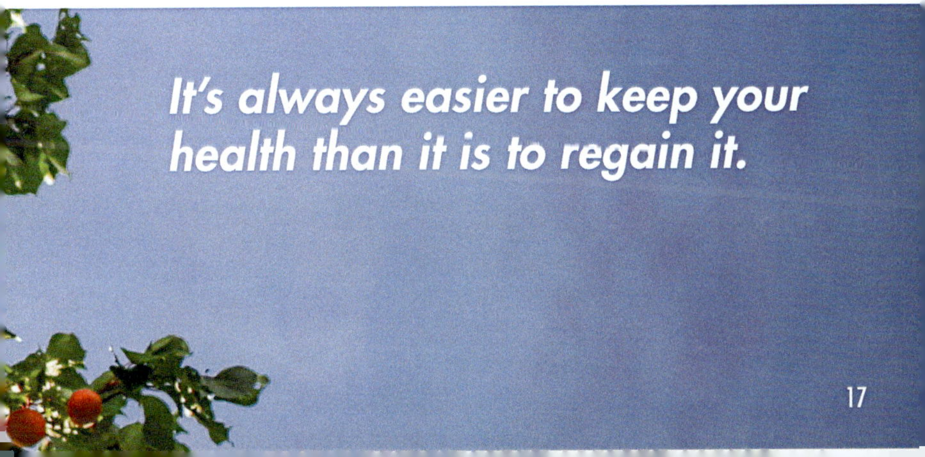

PRACTICE MAKES PERFECT

If you've ever played sports, you can remember the grueling first couple weeks of practice, where the coaches go back to the basics. In football, the coaches focus on blocking, tackling, passing and catching. In basketball, the focus is on free throws, passing and layups. In volleyball, they focus on spikes, blocks, digs and passing.

It doesn't matter if you are new to the game or a seasoned professional: the basics are essential to maintaining and improving your performance.

Just as coaches focus on the basics of their sport, the First21 Challenges focus on the basics of eating, moving and thinking. In order to be healthy, your body and mind will always require gratitude, exercise, water and vegetables, while minimizing sugar, processed foods and chemical additives. Essentially the First21 Challenges are like the practice drills to help you maintain and improve your health in the game of life.

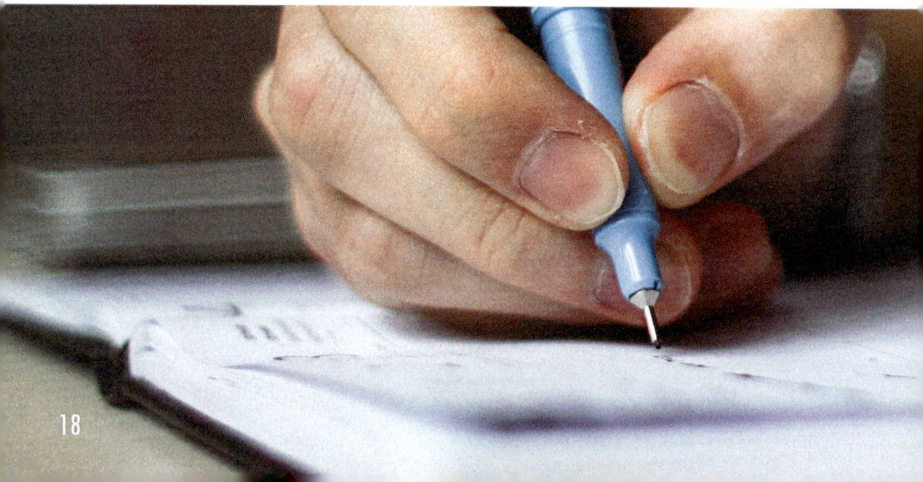

Unlike other diet or fitness challenges, the lessons you learn during the First21 will not be forgotten, because they are not a fad or trend. They are timeless in how they identify common lifestyle problems and address them. They champion the basics of good living.

The First21 Challenges are designed to be revisited, repeated, and mastered. At the end of the book you'll find a chapter in which I discuss what to do after successfully completing these health challenges.

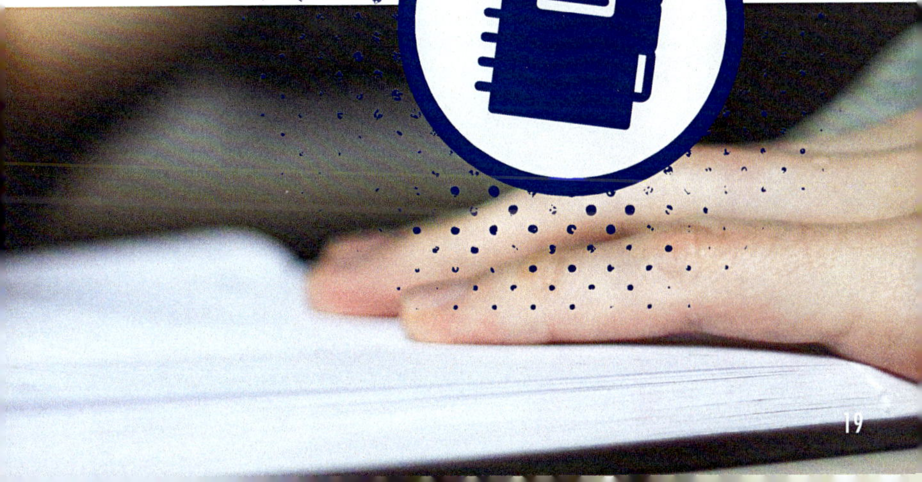

SCHEDULING YOUR JOURNEY

The First21 was designed to be done in small groups, as a corporate wellness program, or even individually with proper guidance. If you are doing the First21 challenges as part of a group, the schedule has been prepared for you. If you are repeating a challenge or doing the challenges individually, you will need to be strategic.

Be sensible about when you start the program. As someone with a sweet tooth, do you really want to embark on your new journey a few days before Halloween? Perhaps there is a food-centric family reunion event you're going to next week. Give yourself a pass, enjoy the event, and start the very next day. Otherwise, you're likely setting yourself up for failure. Review the First21 challenges and schedule them when you will be most successful.

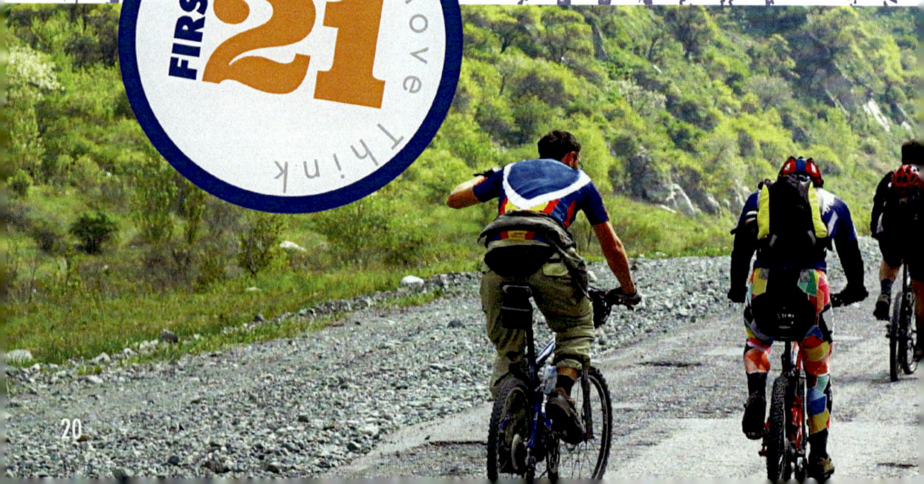

FIRST STEP

In the chapters ahead you will find the First21 challenge overviews and journals. Additional resources for the challenges are located at first21.com. Before starting the First21, it is advised to review your health history and receive a medical release if warranted. Enjoy the journey!

The suggested First21 annual schedule is located in the workbook index.

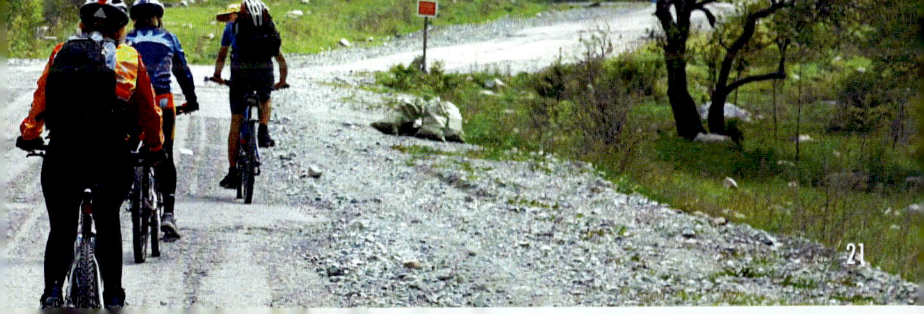

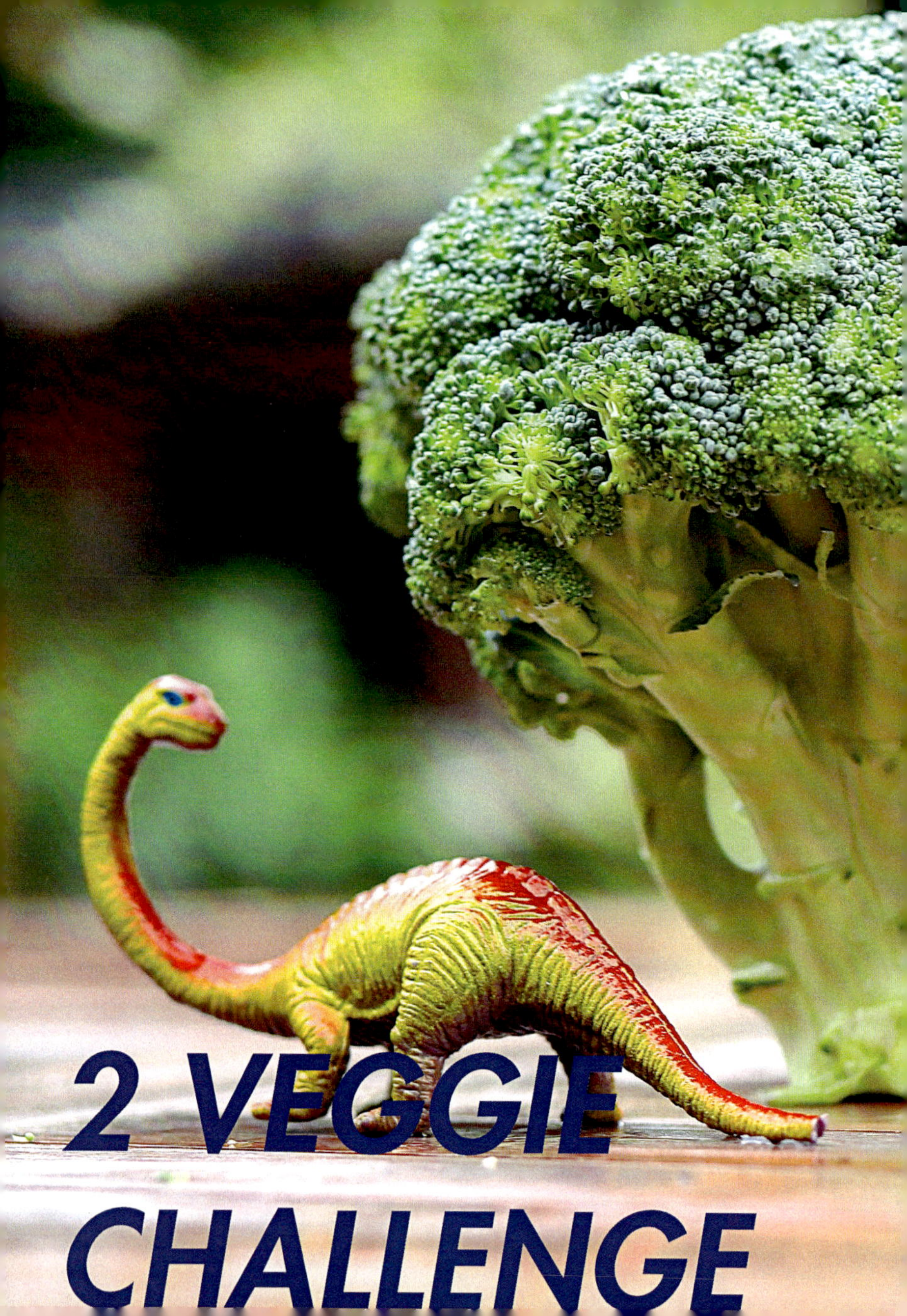

2 VEGGIE CHALLENGE

The stark, green, wholesome truth is your body can't be healthy without eating vegetables.

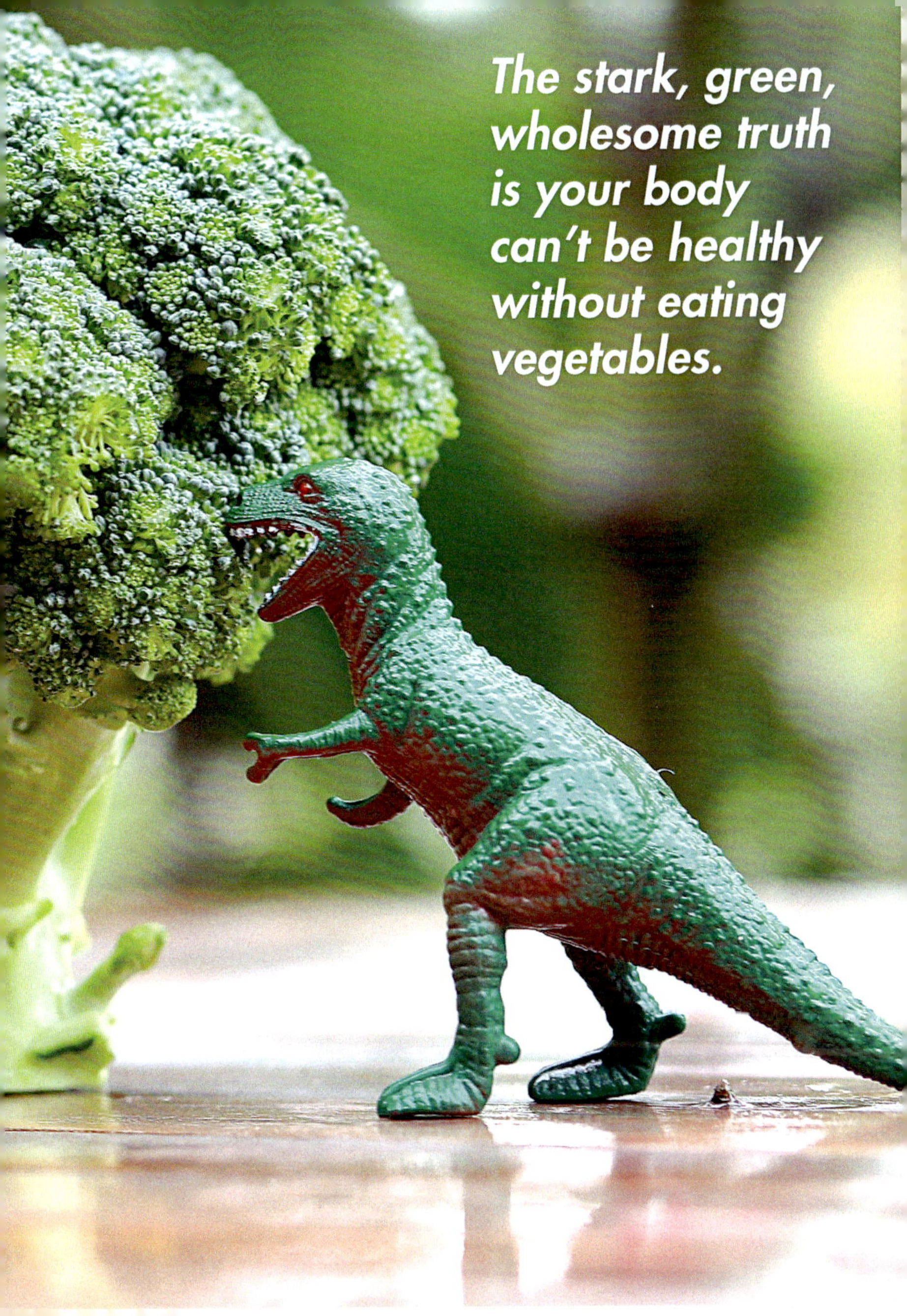

WHY EAT VEGGIES?

If you want to be healthy, vegetables aren't optional. And yet our consumption of them is way too low. Adults in the United States consume vegetables about 1.6 times a day, according to the CDC. Less than a third of the recommended daily intake.

Even more bothersome is how 9 out of 10 children don't eat enough vegetables.

Would it surprise you to learn potatoes and tomatoes are the most commonly consumed vegetables in America? They're *mostly* eaten in the form of French fries and pizza. [7]

The stark, green, wholesome truth is your body can't be healthy without eating vegetables. Here's why:

› They are one of the best sources of antioxidants and are excellent sources of potassium, fiber, folate (folic acid) and vitamins A, E, C. In fact, the nutrients in and benefits of vegetables are as diverse as they look.

› Vegetables can help reduce the risk of heart disease, Type 2 diabetes, obesity, high blood pressure and some cancers. [9,10,11,12,13,14,15]

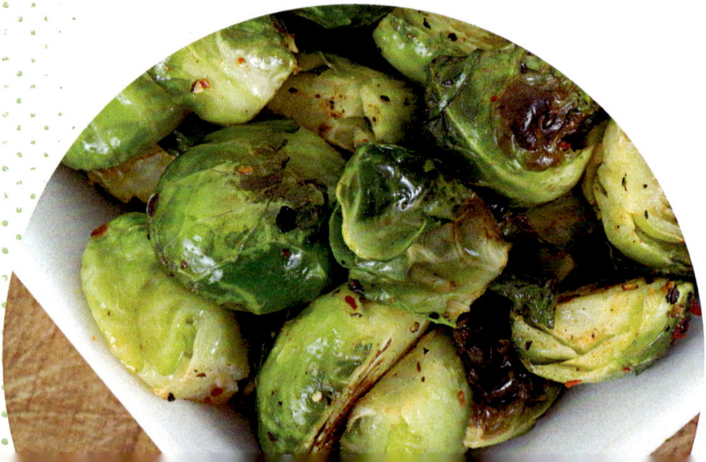

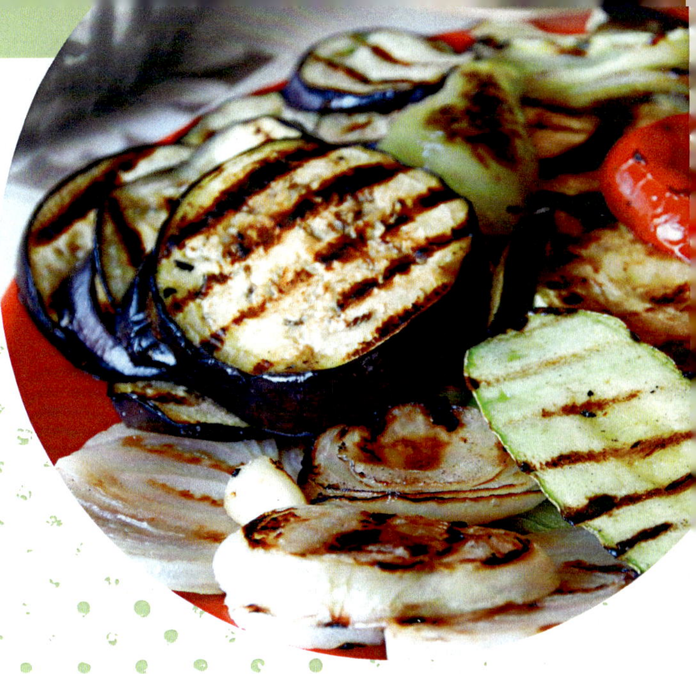

SO HOW MUCH IS ENOUGH?

The USDA recommends 2.5 servings of vegetables a day in order to promote health and decrease your chances of disease, but it's almost impossible to eat too many veggies. [8, 16]

It's the one thing excluded from the moderate category of nutrition because no study yet suggests Americans are sick because they eat too many vegetables. Just be sure to eat a variety because eating any single vegetable over time could lead to nutritional imbalances.

So when it comes to veggies, the more the merrier!

FIRST21 VEGGIE CHALLENGE

Every day for the next 21 days, consume six servings of vegetables. Visit *www.first21.com* for a list of vegetables and serving sizes, plus tips and pointers on how to incorporate more veggies into your diet.

CERTAIN FOODS ARE EXCLUDED FROM THE CHALLENGE.

White Potatoes & Tomatoes

It's clearly not a challenge for Americans to consume these foods. You just have to look at our French fry, potato chip and pizza consumption as proof.

Grains

This includes, but is not limited to, wheat, rice, corn, oats, rye, barley, millet, bulgur, sorghum, buckwheat, sprouted grains, bran, germ and starch.

Legumes

These include black beans, red beans, pinto beans, navy beans, white beans, kidney beans, lima beans, fava beans, chickpeas and lentils. This also includes any bean hummus, peanuts, peanut butter and all forms of soy and soy beans.

Grains and Legumes are commonly mistaken as vegetables. This challenge does not require you to restrict grains and legumes, but they are not to be counted as a serving of vegetables.

(Visit www.first21.com for veggie packed recipes)

Track how many servings of vegetables you eat each day, what they were, and your mood and hunger levels by drawing in facial expressions and the level in the energy gauge.

DATE: Wednesday 7/19 | MOOD | ENERGY

MORNING: spinach, snap peas

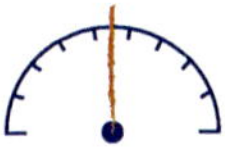

MIDDAY: kale, celery, red pepper

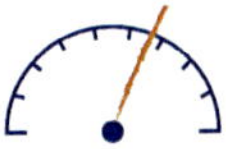

EVENING: cauliflower, spinach

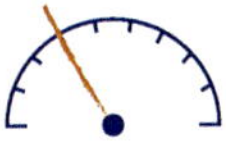

DATE: | MOOD | ENERGY

MORNING:

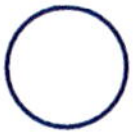
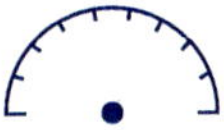

MIDDAY:

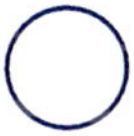
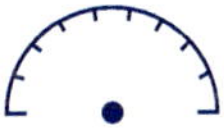

EVENING:

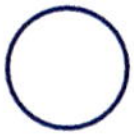
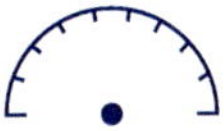

2

DATE:

MOOD ENERGY

MORNING:

MIDDAY:

EVENING:

3

DATE:

MOOD ENERGY

MORNING:

MIDDAY:

EVENING:

DATE: MOOD ENERGY

MORNING:

MIDDAY:

EVENING:

DATE: MOOD ENERGY

MORNING:

MIDDAY:

EVENING:

6

DATE: MOOD ENERGY

MORNING:

MIDDAY:

EVENING:

7

DATE: MOOD ENERGY

MORNING:

MIDDAY:

EVENING:

DATE: MOOD ENERGY

MORNING:

MIDDAY:

EVENING:

DATE: MOOD ENERGY

MORNING:

MIDDAY:

EVENING:

DATE: MOOD ENERGY

MORNING:

MIDDAY:

EVENING:

10

DATE: MOOD ENERGY

MORNING:

MIDDAY:

EVENING:

11

DATE: MOOD ENERGY

MORNING:

MIDDAY:

EVENING:

12

DATE: MOOD ENERGY

MORNING:

MIDDAY:

EVENING:

13

14

DATE: MOOD ENERGY

MORNING:

MIDDAY:

EVENING:

15

DATE: MOOD ENERGY

MORNING:

MIDDAY:

EVENING:

DATE: MOOD ENERGY

MORNING:

MIDDAY:

EVENING:

DATE: MOOD ENERGY

MORNING:

MIDDAY:

EVENING:

DATE: | MOOD | ENERGY

MORNING:

MIDDAY:

EVENING:

18

DATE: | MOOD | ENERGY

MORNING:

MIDDAY:

EVENING:

19

DATE: MOOD ENERGY

MORNING:

MIDDAY:

EVENING:

DATE: MOOD ENERGY

MORNING:

MIDDAY:

EVENING:

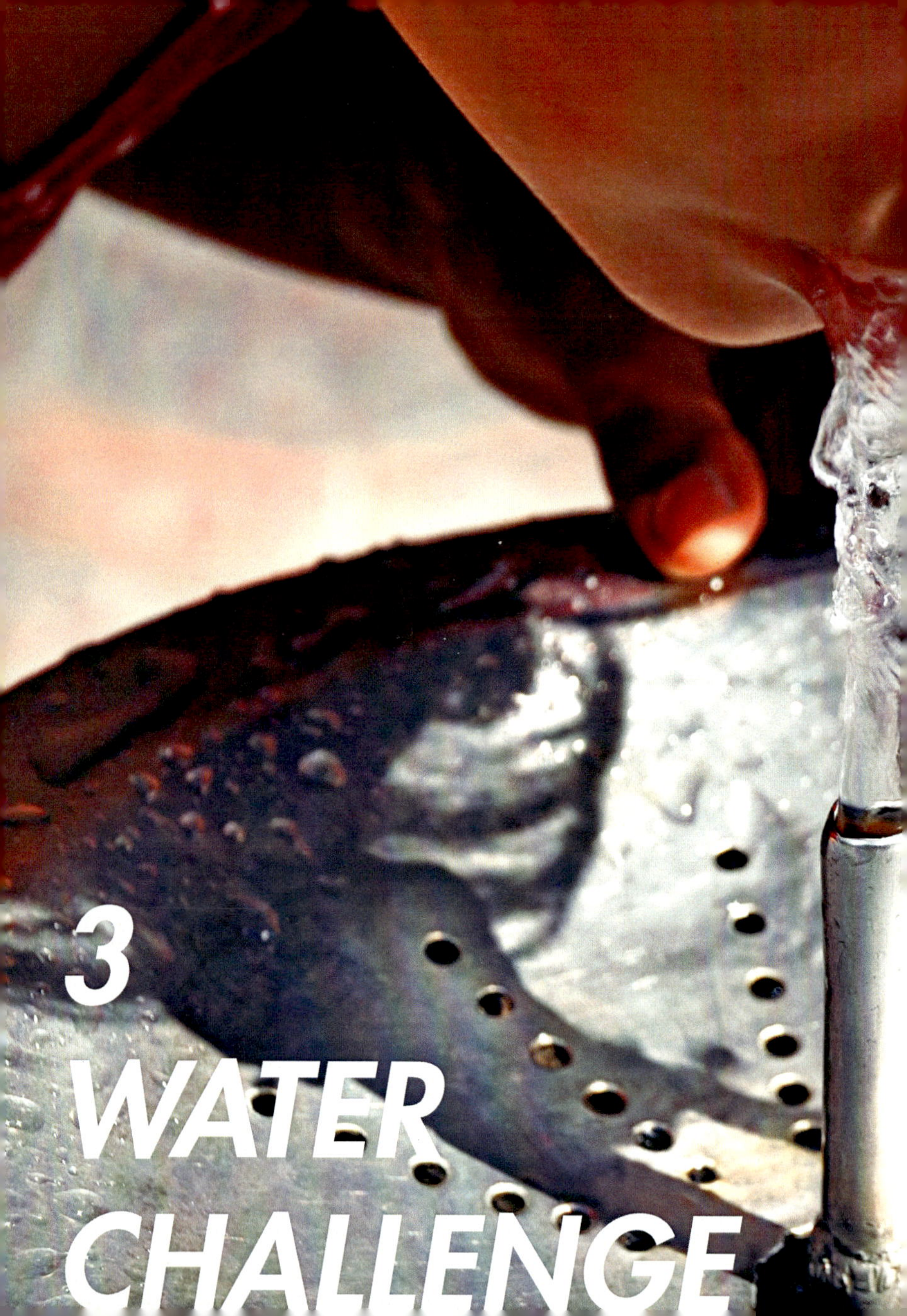

3 WATER CHALLENGE

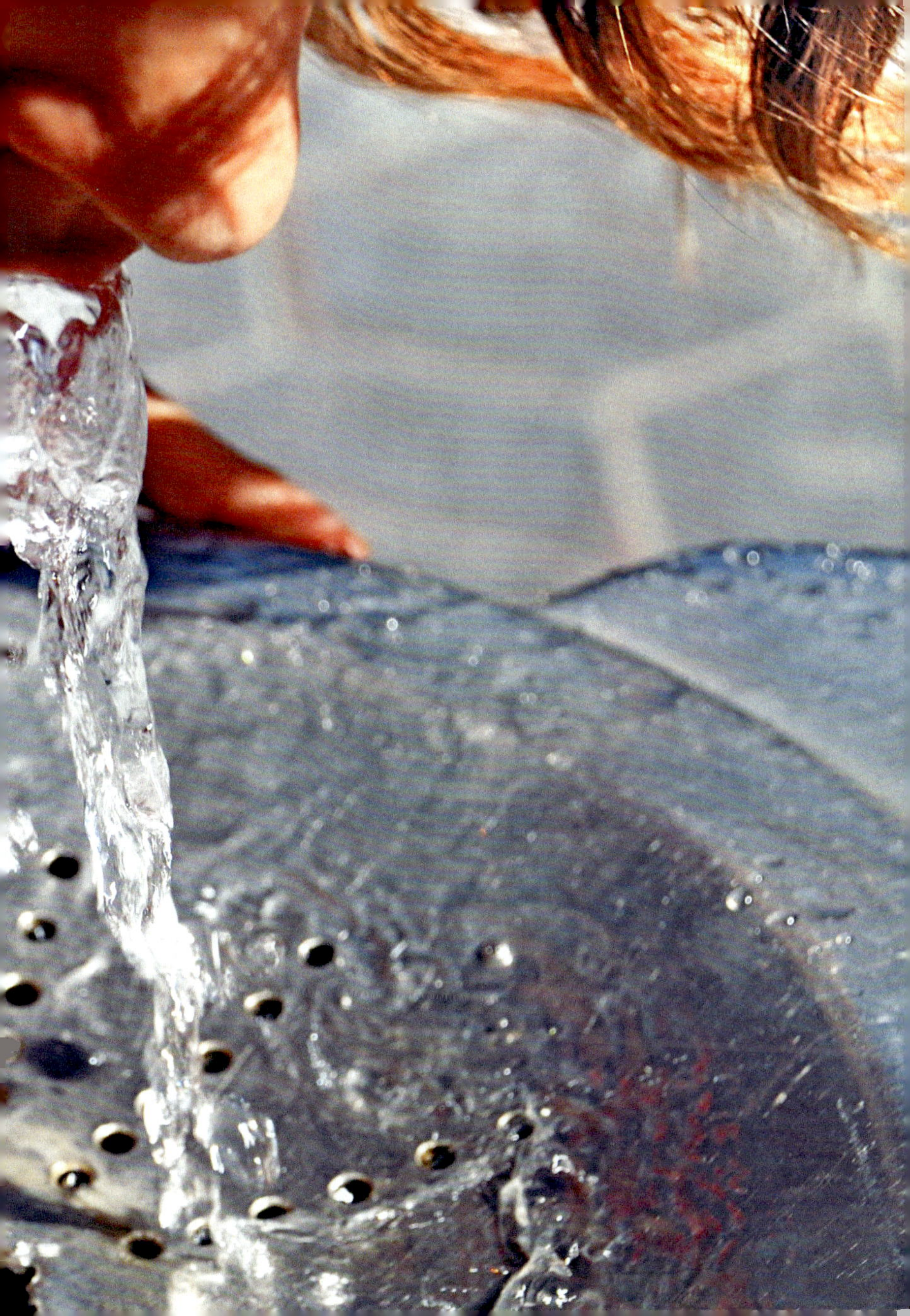

Drinking water can vastly improve your general health

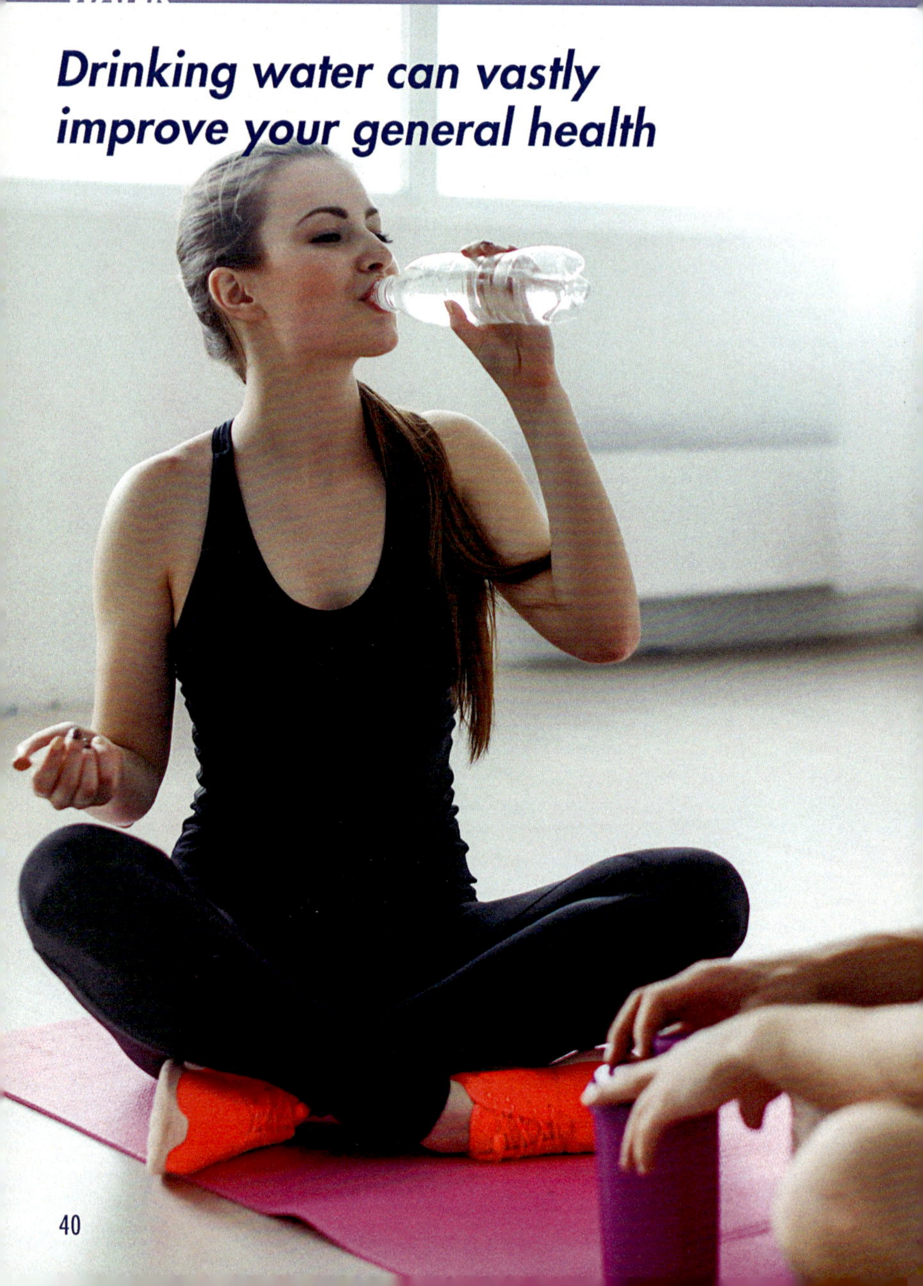

WHY DRINK WATER?

Every cell, tissue, and organ in your body requires water to function optimally. Water is also one of the body's most important cleaning tools. If you drink more "other" drinks than you do water, it's like washing your dishes with dirty water.

Drinking water is great for your skin and joints, but it can also vastly improve your general health. Here's what water does for you: [17]

- ***Regulates body temperature***
- ***Cushions and lubricates your joints***
- ***Protects sensitive tissues like your nervous system***
- ***Removes waste through urination, perspiration and bowel movements***

TIRED? MOODY? MAYBE YOU'RE DEHYDRATED

Feeling a little crazy today? Research has shown mild dehydration can cause mood swings and problems with concentration. In the same research they found it didn't matter if the person was sitting at a desk or exercising on a treadmill – either way, they were just as likely to feel the effects of mild dehydration. [18, 19, 20] Simply drinking too many diuretic drinks like alcohol, coffee and black tea can cause your body to urinate frequently and lead to dehydration. Here are the signs: [21]

- ***Thirst***
- ***Dry and/or sticky mouth***
- ***Fatigue***
- ***Sleepiness (Children may be less active than normal)***
- ***Decreased urine output***
- ***Headache***
- ***Difficulty concentrating***
- ***Dizziness or lightheadedness***

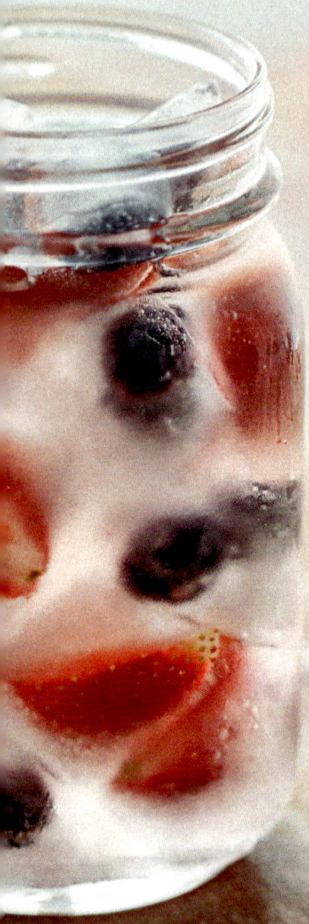

FIRST21 WATER CHALLENGE

There is no exact 'science' when it comes to water consumption. It varies according to our weight, activity level, the climate, and where in the world we live. The First21 Water Challenge recommendation is to at least consume half of your body weight in ounces each day for the next 21 days. So if you weigh 160 pounds, you'll be drinking 80 ounces of water – five pints. If you consume any diuretic drinks, such as alcohol, coffee or black tea, consume an equivalent in additional ounces of water.

To keep track of your water consumption (or lack of it!) we advise journaling all beverages consumed in the First21 Water Challenge Journal.

How much water should you consume?

Body Weight/2= ________ oz

Journal the beverages you consume each day by filling in a glass icon for every 12 ounces. Write what you drank below the glass and the size of your glass if it is larger or smaller than 12 ounces. Draw a line to indicate your daily goal.

DATE: Tuesday 5/17

TOTAL:
120 oz

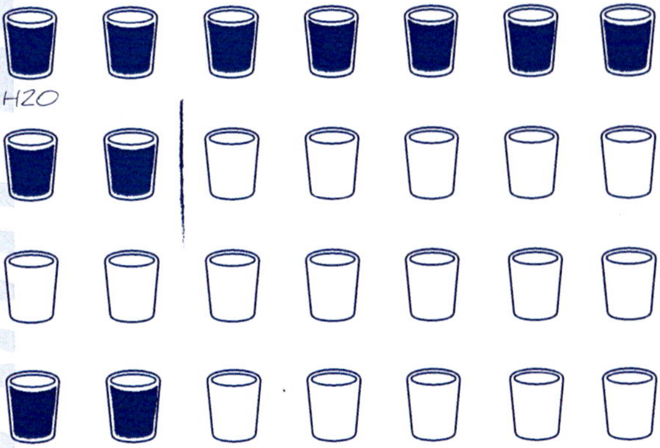

DIURETICS:

TOTAL:
24 oz

DAY'S TOTAL: 120 oz water - 24 oz diuretics = 96 oz

1

DATE:

TOTAL:

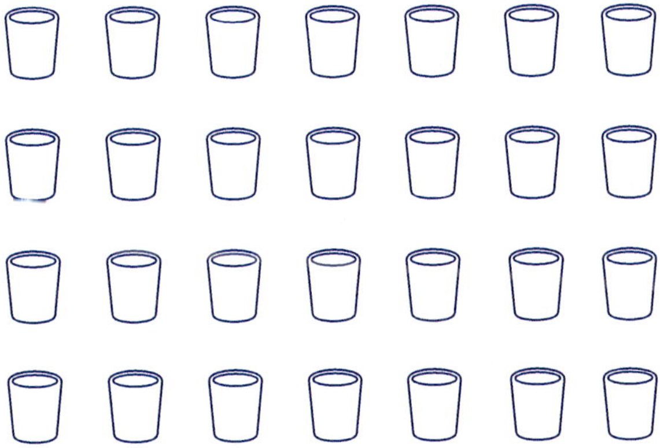

DIURETICS:

TOTAL:

DAY'S TOTAL:

DATE:

TOTAL:

DIURETICS:

TOTAL:

DAY'S TOTAL:

2

DATE:

TOTAL:

DIURETICS:

TOTAL:

DAY'S TOTAL:

3

DATE:

TOTAL:

DIURETICS:

TOTAL:

DAY'S TOTAL:

DATE:

TOTAL:

DIURETICS:

TOTAL:

DAY'S TOTAL:

DATE:

TOTAL:

DIURETICS:

TOTAL:

DAY'S TOTAL:

DATE:

TOTAL:

DIURETICS:

TOTAL:

DAY'S TOTAL:

8

DATE:

TOTAL:

DIURETICS:

TOTAL:

DAY'S TOTAL:

9

DATE:

TOTAL:

DIURETICS:

TOTAL:

DAY'S TOTAL:

10

DATE:

TOTAL:

DIURETICS:

TOTAL:

DAY'S TOTAL:

11

DATE:

TOTAL:

DIURETICS:

TOTAL:

DAY'S TOTAL:

12

DATE:

TOTAL:

DIURETICS:

TOTAL:

DAY'S TOTAL:

13

DATE:

TOTAL:

DIURETICS:

TOTAL:

DAY'S TOTAL:

14

DATE:

TOTAL:

DIURETICS:

TOTAL:

DAY'S TOTAL:

15

DATE:

TOTAL:

DIURETICS:

TOTAL:

DAY'S TOTAL:

16

DATE:

TOTAL:

DIURETICS:

TOTAL:

DAY'S TOTAL:

17

DATE:

TOTAL:

DIURETICS:

TOTAL:

DAY'S TOTAL:

18

DATE:

TOTAL:

DIURETICS:

TOTAL:

DAY'S TOTAL:

19

DATE:

TOTAL:

DIURETICS:

TOTAL:

DAY'S TOTAL:

20

DATE:

TOTAL:

DIURETICS:

TOTAL:

DAY'S TOTAL:

21

DATE:

TOTAL:

DIURETICS:

TOTAL:

DAY'S TOTAL:

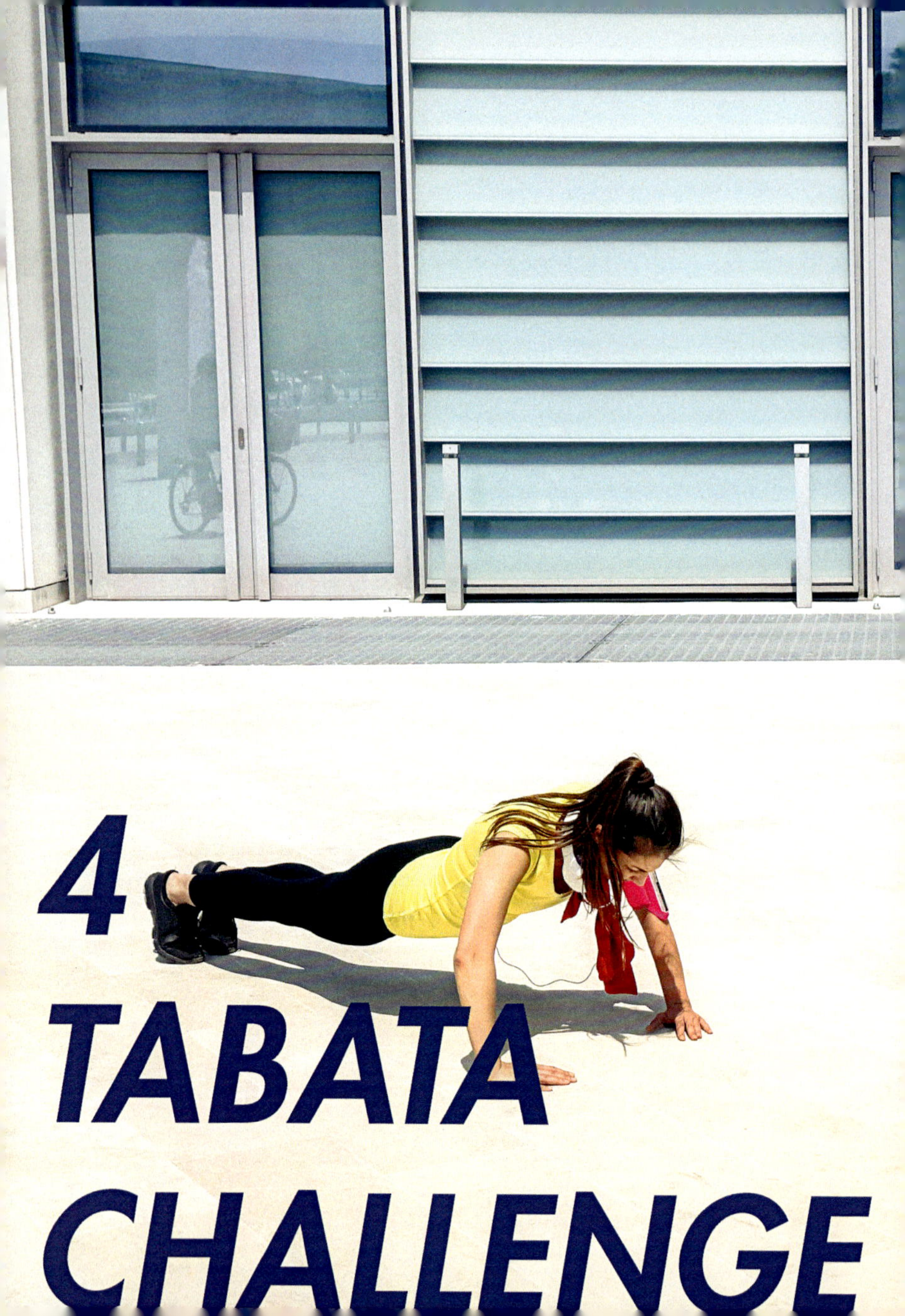

4 TABATA CHALLENGE

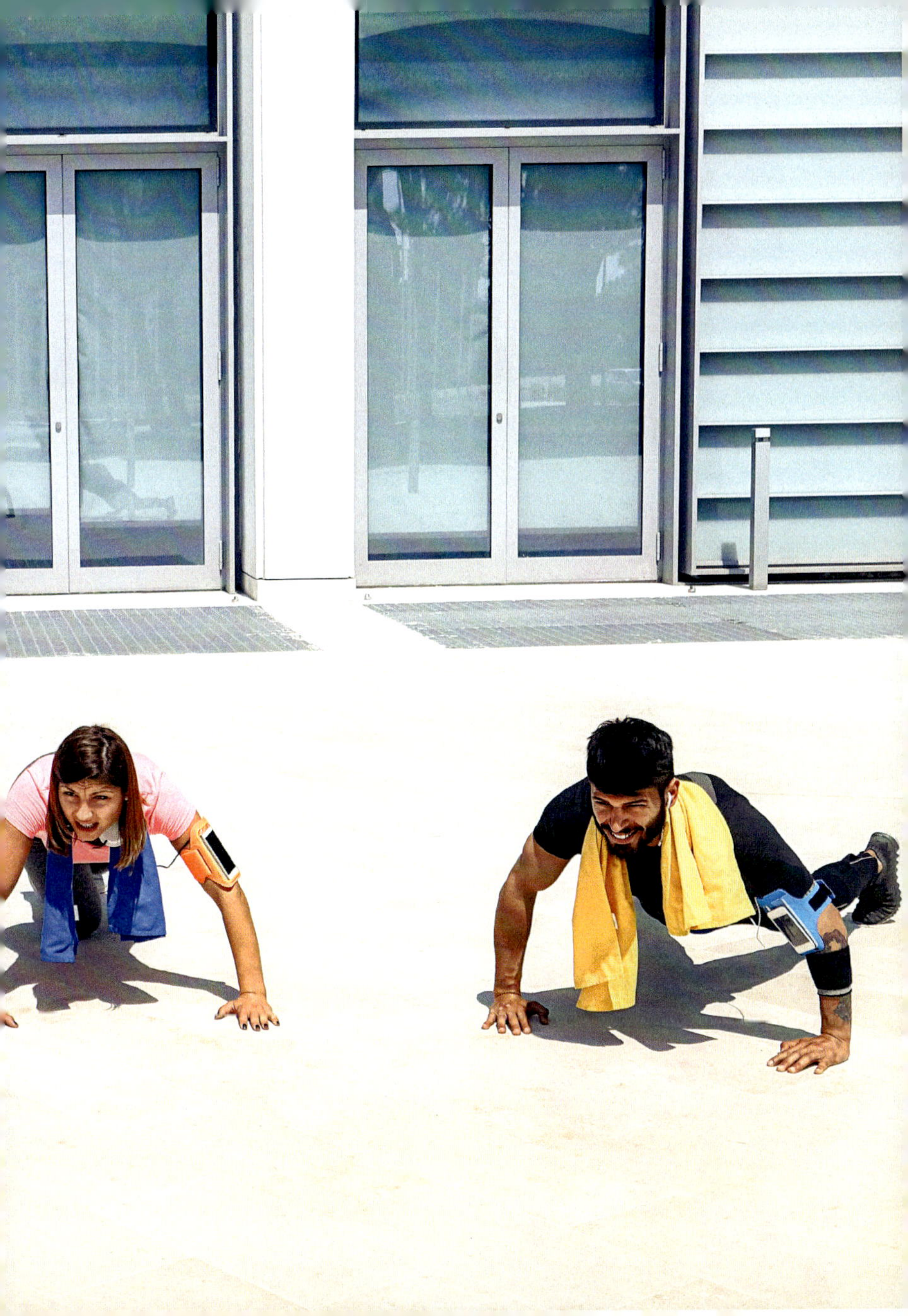

NO TIME FOR EXERCISE? HERE'S YOUR SOLUTION

Fact is, it's easy to sign up for the gym, but it's not always easy to get there.

Life is busy. After a long day most of us don't have enough energy to drive 15 minutes to the gym, exercise for 60 minutes on a treadmill, then drive 15 minutes back home. In reality, by the time you add in a quick shower, about 2 hours of the day are gone.

When it comes to exercise, most of us need something quick, repeatable and systematic in order to be successful. The First21 Tabata Challenge includes a dynamic warm-up, functional exercise, and cool down stretches to be done at home, on the go, or under a trainer's supervision.

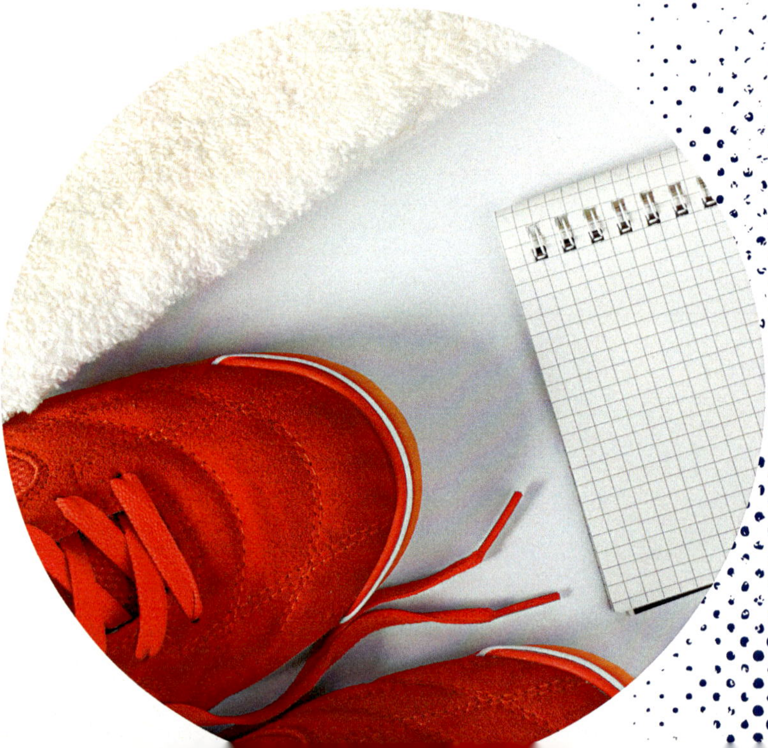

WHAT IS TABATA?

First, it is important to understand a Tabata is not a movement. Instead, a Tabata is a form of high intensity interval training. Each Tabata is performed by doing 20 seconds of work followed by 10 seconds of rest, repeated for a total of 8 cycles. You will be keeping score on one movement for each 4-minute Tabata, which will allow you to monitor the progression of your strength and endurance.

Amazingly, the scalability of the Tabata challenge is what makes it so doable! You may not be able to do a push-up from your toes, but you can probably do a push-up from your knees or against a wall. In fact, any healthy functional movement can be performed as a Tabata exercise to improve joint stability, strength, endurance and balance.

(Visit www.first21.com for a tabata clock)

HOW TO KEEP SCORE

If you are doing a movement requiring you to hold one position for as long as you can, your score for the Tabata will be the total seconds held in position after 8 rounds. An example would be holding steady in a plank.

If you are doing a movement requiring you to do repetitions, your score for the Tabata will be the total repetitions completed after all 8 rounds. An example would be the number of squats completed.

WHY IS IT CALLED A TABATA?

In 1996, Dr. Izumi Tabata collaborated with the Japanese speed skating team to determine an optimum training protocol. His research compared two groups of athletes, exercising 5 days a week for 6 weeks. The first group performed a Tabata protocol including a 5-minute warm up, a 4-minute Tabata, and a 5-minute cool down, for a total exercise time of 14 minutes. The second group ran at 70% of their effort for a total of 60 minutes. As a result, the athletes practicing Tabata lost body fat without losing muscle mass, improved their aerobic capacity by 14% and their anaerobic capacity by 28%, compared to the traditional running protocol athletes, which showed only a 9.5% improvement in their aerobic or endurance capacity and no effect on their anaerobic capacity, which relates to brief, high-intensity exercise. [22]

Simply put, Tabata exercise protocols are perfect for people who want great results with minimal time invested!

LISTEN TO YOUR BODY

Taking action is the most important part of the First21. On your first Tabata, use only 50% of your full effort. Only increase your intensity as you feel more comfortable.

It is easy to underestimate how difficult 8 cycles of any exercise may be.

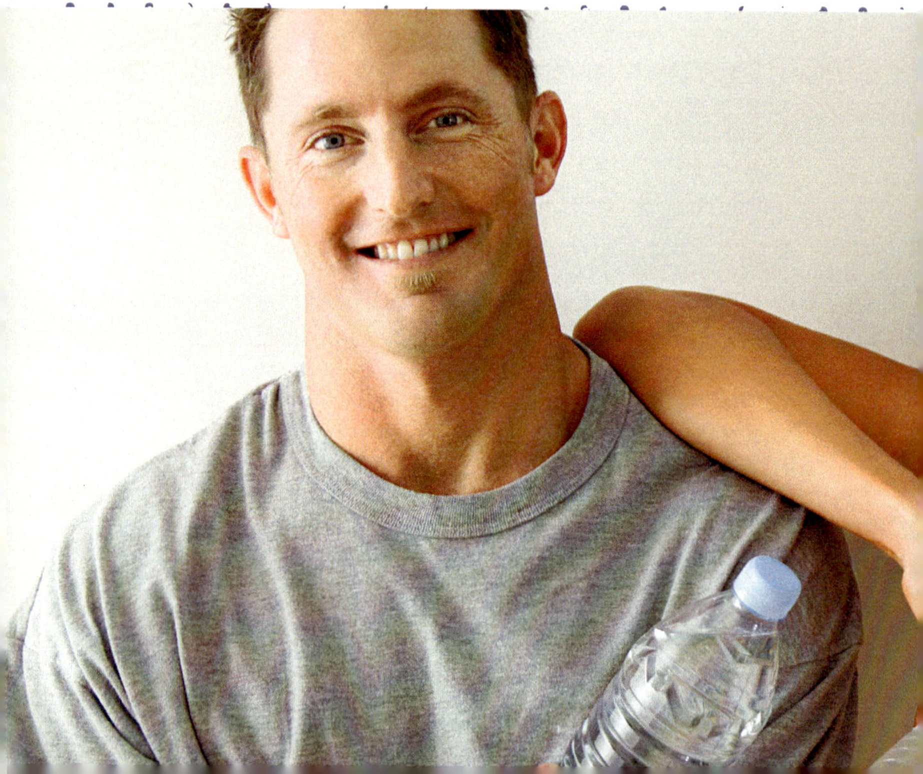

As an example, if you were performing a Tabata of sprints, you would only lightly jog. This will allow you to use healthy functional movement, and ensures you do not over-exert yourself the first time out. There is no glory in NOT working out tomorrow. Do less reps, go at a slower pace and make things harder with time.

Remember, you are the boss of your body but you must listen to what it's saying. Do not exercise beyond your current level of health and fitness. The First21 is meant to be your starting point, not your ending point.

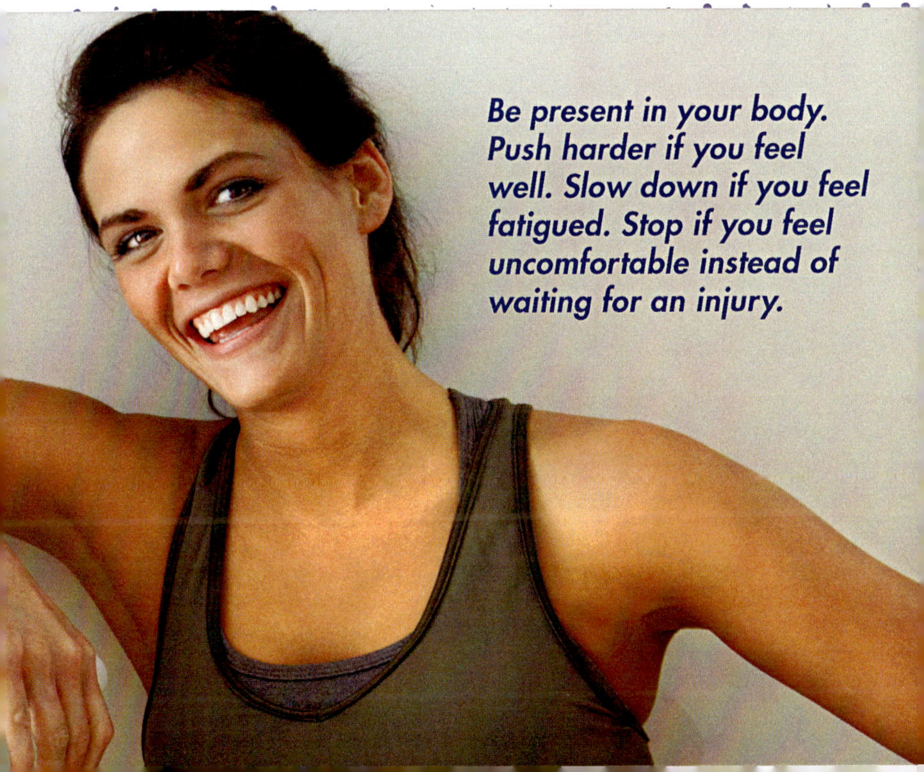

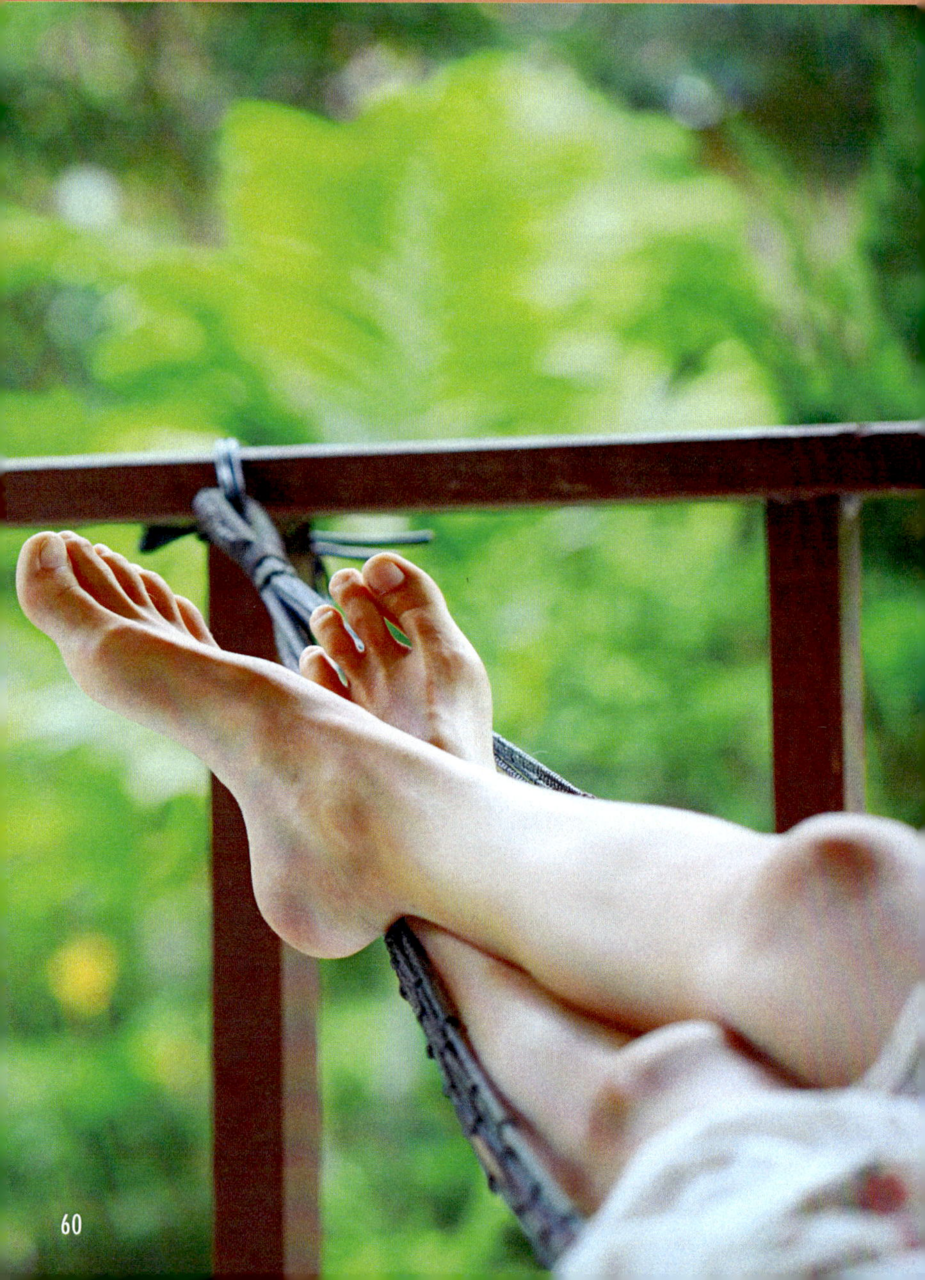

REMEMBER:

- *Visit your doctor for a full medical check-up before starting any exercise program*
- *Respect your current fitness level by starting an exercise program at a pace you can maintain*
- *Injuries require rest and recovery. Working through pain will only cause more damage and delay healing*
- *If you have a pre-existing injury or are prone to injury, consult your doctor before starting any exercise program*

STOP EXERCISING AND SEEK MEDICAL HELP IF YOU EXPERIENCE ANY OF THE FOLLOWING SYMPTOMS:

- *You feel pain or discomfort*
- *You feel chest pain that could indicate a heart attack, including pain in the neck, jaw, pain traveling down the arm or pain between the shoulder blades*
- *You experience any breathlessness or inability to catch your breath*
- *You develop a rapid or irregular heartbeat during exercise*
- *You experience joint pain persisting after more than three days of rest*

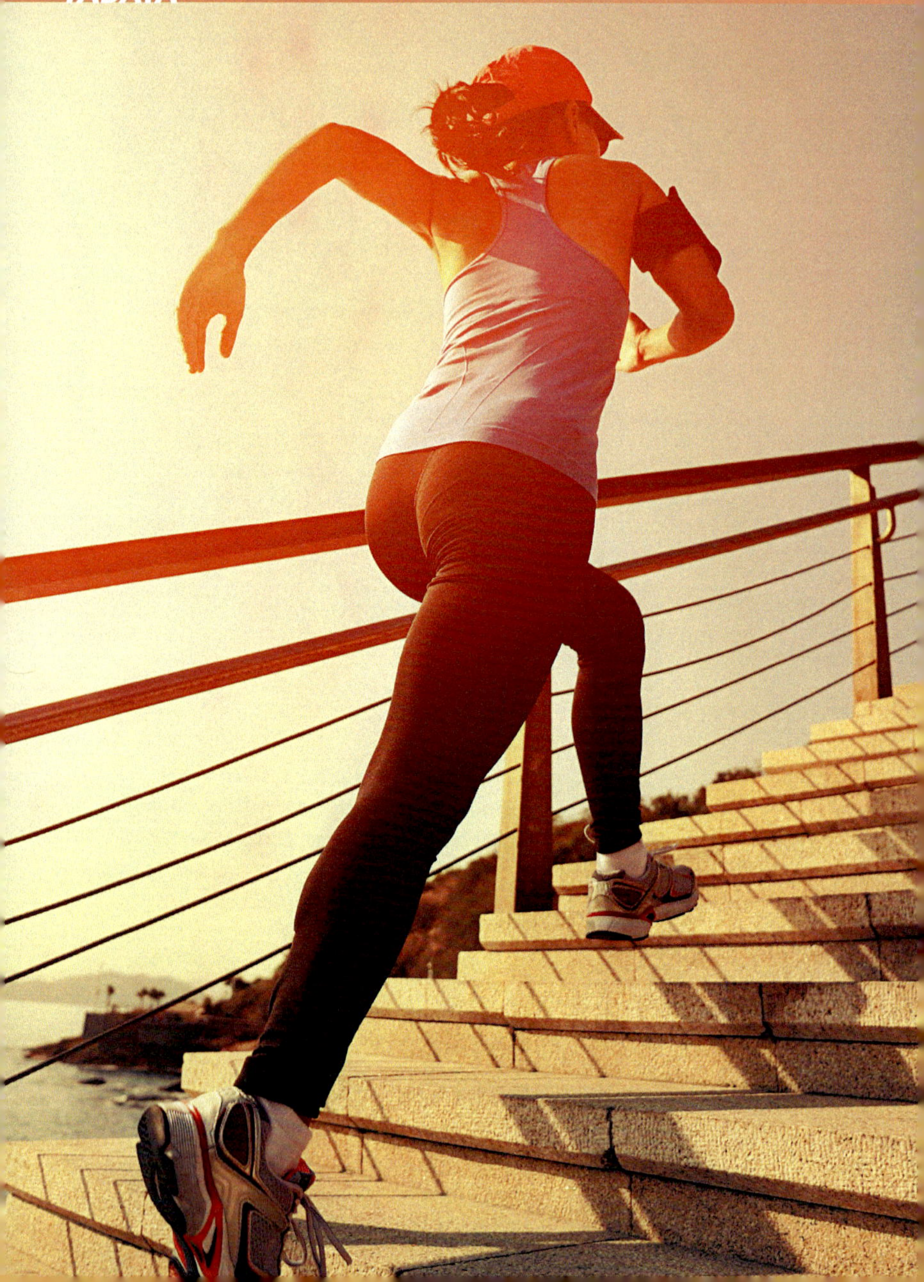

AT WHAT LEVEL SHOULD YOU START?

The Tabata Challenge is programed for the intermediate level athlete. If you are new to exercise and high intensity interval training it will be important for you to use the beginner modifications. Experienced athletes can use the advanced modifications to intensify their challenge. Additional exercises are located at ***first21.com.***

Answering the following questions will help decide which level you should start with. Circle "YES" or "NO" to the following questions:

YES / NO	Are you interested in being healthier?
YES / NO	Are you interested in becoming stronger?
YES / NO	Currently, can you can exercise with NO limitations?
YES / NO	Can you walk up stairs without shortness of breath?
YES / NO	Have you ever participated in a Tabata or High Intensity Interval Training Workout?
YES / NO	Have you exercised consistently for 3 or more days per week for the past 6 months?
YES / NO	When you exercise, does your intensity level raise your respiration and heart rate?
YES / NO	Can you do 20 standard pushups unbroken?
YES / NO	Can you do 50 consecutive air squats unbroken?
YES / NO	Can you hold a 2 minute Plank with a flat back?

________How many "YES" answers did you have?

The total number of YES answers to indicate which level is best for you.

If you answered YES to 1-4 questions, start with the beginner programming.
If you answered YES to 5-9 questions, start with the intermediate programming.
If you answered YES to 10 questions, start with the advanced programming.

HOW TO BEGIN

Each daily journal entry has the recommended movement to be performed. In addition you will need to do a 4 minute warm up before your Tabata and cool down stretches following your Tabata. On rest days you will only perform the 4 minute warm up followed by the cool down stretches.

There is a full video catalog of exercises located at www.first21.com. If you are uncomfortable or unable to perform a recommended movement it can be exchanged with a more manageable movement from the video catalog located on the first21 website.

Unable to do the Tabata challenge because of an injury or your current level of health? **Consider doing the Walking Challenge instead!**

QUICK REFERENCE

WARM UP

20	10	8
seconds of any movement	seconds of rest	cycles of repetitions

----

COOL DOWN STRETCHES

Visit www.first21.com for a complete catalogue of movements and a timer.

4 MINUTE WARM UP

Perform each movement for 30 seconds and repeat one time. Advanced 4 Minute Warm Up at www.first21.com.

1. MARCH IN PLACE (Constant movement)

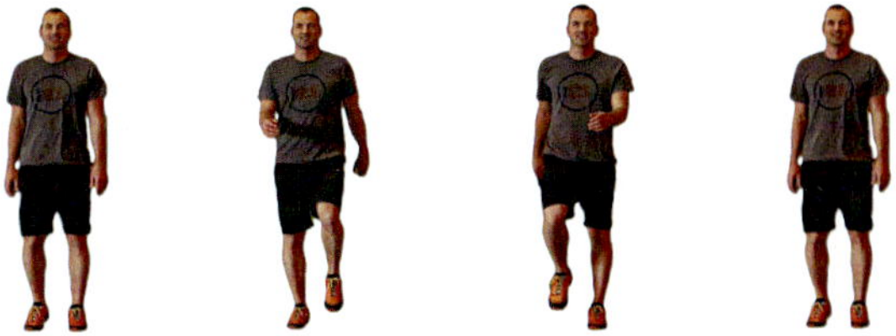

2. FORWARD BENDS (Constant movement)

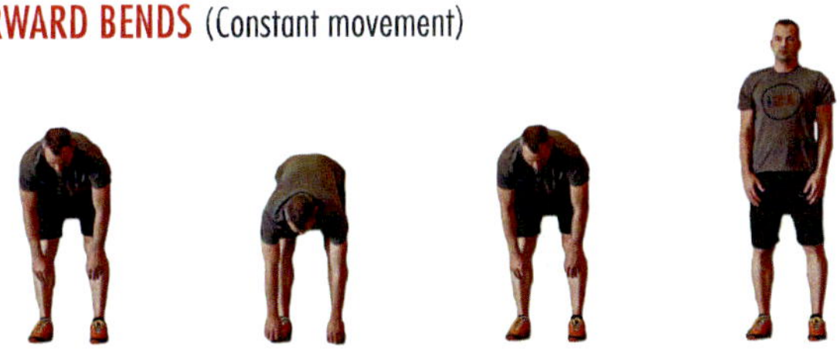

3. KNEE TUCK (Constant movement)

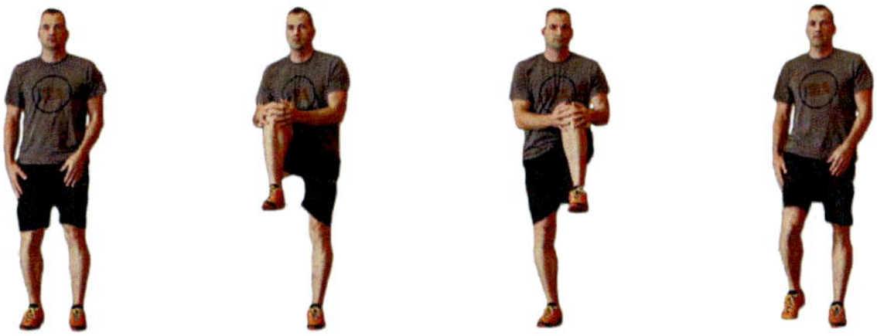

4. SIDE STEP WITH BACK TAP (Constant movement)

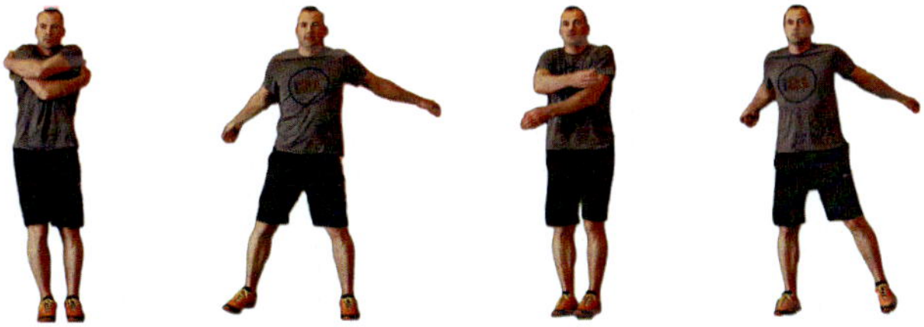

7 MINUTE COOL DOWN STRETCH 4 sets of 10 second holds

1. FORWARD BEND (TOE TOUCH)

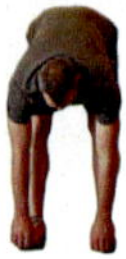

2. LUNGE STRETCH

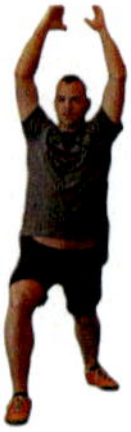

3. KNEE HUG

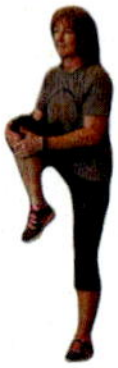

4. SEATED GLUTEAL STRETCH

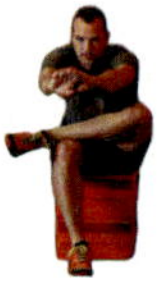

5. TRICEPS STRETCH

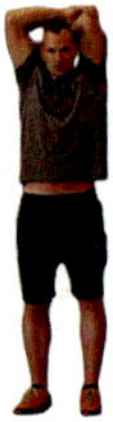

6. CROSS BODY STRETCH

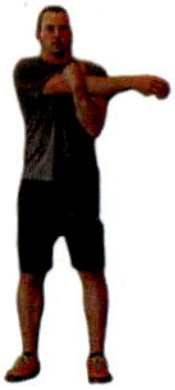

7. WALL STRETCH

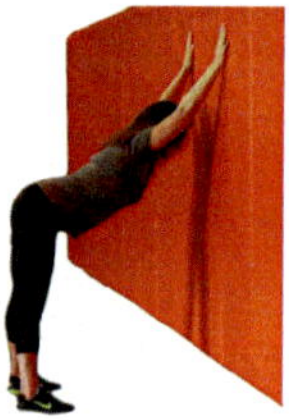

Visit www.first21.com for example videos of each movement

Journal your tabata sessions. Your score is the total repetitions completed during four minutes.

WARM UP » **20** SECONDS OF DAY'S MOVEMENT » **10** SECONDS OF REST »
8 CYCLES OF REPETITIONS » **COOL DOWN STRETCHES**

SAMPLE

DATE: Mon, 3/04 MOVEMENT: BURPEES

CYCLE 1: 8 CYCLE 2: 10 CYCLE 3: 11

CYCLE 4: 9 CYCLE 5: 5 CYCLE 6: 13

CYCLE 7: 11 CYCLE 8: 9 TOTAL POINTS: 76

1

DATE: MOVEMENT: BIRD DOG

CYCLE 1: CYCLE 2: CYCLE 3:

CYCLE 4: CYCLE 5: CYCLE 6:

CYCLE 7: CYCLE 8: TOTAL POINTS:

2

DATE: MOVEMENT: ACTIVE REST DAY

PERFORM THE WARM UP AND COOL DOWN STRETCHES

WARM UP » **20** SECONDS OF DAY'S MOVEMENT » **10** SECONDS OF REST » **8** CYCLES OF REPETITIONS » **COOL DOWN STRETCHES**

3

DATE: MOVEMENT: STANDING BICYCLES

CYCLE 1: CYCLE 2: CYCLE 3:

CYCLE 4: CYCLE 5: CYCLE 6:

CYCLE 7: CYCLE 8: TOTAL POINTS:

4

DATE: MOVEMENT: ACTIVE REST DAY

PERFORM THE WARM UP AND COOL DOWN STRETCHES

5

DATE: MOVEMENT: AIR SQUAT – BEGINNER: CHAIR SIT
ADVANCED: OVERHEAD SQUAT

CYCLE 1: CYCLE 2: CYCLE 3:

CYCLE 4: CYCLE 5: CYCLE 6:

CYCLE 7: CYCLE 8: TOTAL POINTS:

(Visit www.first21.com for example videos of each movement)

DATE: MOVEMENT: REVERSE FLUTTER KICKS

6

CYCLE 1:	CYCLE 2:	CYCLE 3:
CYCLE 4:	CYCLE 5:	CYCLE 6:
CYCLE 7:	CYCLE 8:	TOTAL POINTS:

DATE: MOVEMENT: ACTIVE REST DAY

7

PERFORM THE WARM UP AND COOL DOWN STRETCHES

DATE: MOVEMENT: PLANK – BEGINNER: KNEE PLANK
ADVANCED: PLANK PYRAMIDS

8

CYCLE 1:	CYCLE 2:	CYCLE 3.
CYCLE 4:	CYCLE 5:	CYCLE 6:
CYCLE 7:	CYCLE 8:	TOTAL POINTS:

WARM UP » **20** SECONDS OF DAY'S MOVEMENT » **10** SECONDS OF REST » **8** CYCLES OF REPETITIONS » **COOL DOWN STRETCHES**

9

DATE:

MOVEMENT: GLUTEAL BRIDGE HANDS DOWN

CYCLE 1: CYCLE 2: CYCLE 3:

CYCLE 4: CYCLE 5: CYCLE 6:

CYCLE 7: CYCLE 8: TOTAL POINTS:

10

DATE:

MOVEMENT: ACTIVE REST DAY

PERFORM THE WARM UP AND COOL DOWN STRETCHES

11

DATE:

MOVEMENT: SUPERMAN
ADVANCED: SUPERMAN PRESS PLANK

CYCLE 1: CYCLE 2: CYCLE 3:

CYCLE 4: CYCLE 5: CYCLE 6:

CYCLE 7: CYCLE 8: TOTAL POINTS:

(Visit www.first21.com for example videos of each movement)

12

DATE:

MOVEMENT: FLUTTER KICKS
ADVANCED: SUPERMAN FLUTTER KICKS

CYCLE 1: CYCLE 2: CYCLE 3:

CYCLE 4: CYCLE 5: CYCLE 6:

CYCLE 7: CYCLE 8: TOTAL POINTS:

13

DATE:

MOVEMENT: ACTIVE REST DAY

PERFORM THE WARM UP AND COOL DOWN STRETCHES

14

DATE:

MOVEMENT: MOUNTAIN CLIMBERS – BEGINNER: MARCHING HIGH KNEES
ADVANCED: KNEE TO ELBOW MOUNTAIN CLIMBERS

CYCLE 1: CYCLE 2: CYCLE 3:

CYCLE 4: CYCLE 5: CYCLE 6:

CYCLE 7: CYCLE 8: TOTAL POINTS:

WARM UP » 20 SECONDS OF DAY'S MOVEMENT **» 10** SECONDS OF REST »
8 CYCLES OF REPETITIONS » **COOL DOWN STRETCHES**

15

DATE: MOVEMENT: PLANK – BEGINNER: KNEE PLANK (SECONDS HELD)
ADVANCED: PLANK PYRAMIDS (REPETITIONS)

CYCLE 1: CYCLE 2: CYCLE 3:

CYCLE 4: CYCLE 5: CYCLE 6:

CYCLE 7: CYCLE 8: TOTAL POINTS:

16

DATE: MOVEMENT: ACTIVE REST DAY

PERFORM THE WARM UP AND COOL DOWN STRETCHES

17

DATE: MOVEMENT: LEGS ONLY HALF BICYCLES

CYCLE 1: CYCLE 2: CYCLE 3:

CYCLE 4: CYCLE 5: CYCLE 6:

CYCLE 7: CYCLE 8: TOTAL POINTS:

(Visit www.first21.com for example videos of each movement)

18

DATE: MOVEMENT: BIRD DOG

CYCLE 1: CYCLE 2: CYCLE 3:

CYCLE 4: CYCLE 5: CYCLE 6:

CYCLE 7: CYCLE 8: TOTAL POINTS:

19

DATE: MOVEMENT: ACTIVE REST DAY

PERFORM THE WARM UP AND COOL DOWN STRETCHES

20

DATE: MOVEMENT: CONTROLLED CALF RAISES

CYCLE 1: CYCLE 2: CYCLE 3:

CYCLE 4: CYCLE 5: CYCLE 6:

CYCLE 7: CYCLE 8: TOTAL POINTS:

WARM UP » **20** SECONDS OF DAY'S MOVEMENT » **10** SECONDS OF REST »
8 CYCLES OF REPETITIONS » **COOL DOWN STRETCHES**

DATE:

MOVEMENT: SQUAT – BEGINNER: CHAIR SIT
ADVANCED: OVERHEAD SQUAT

CYCLE 1:

CYCLE 2:

CYCLE 3:

CYCLE 4:

CYCLE 5:

CYCLE 6:

CYCLE 7:

CYCLE 8:

TOTAL POINTS:

(Visit www.first21.com for example videos of each movement)

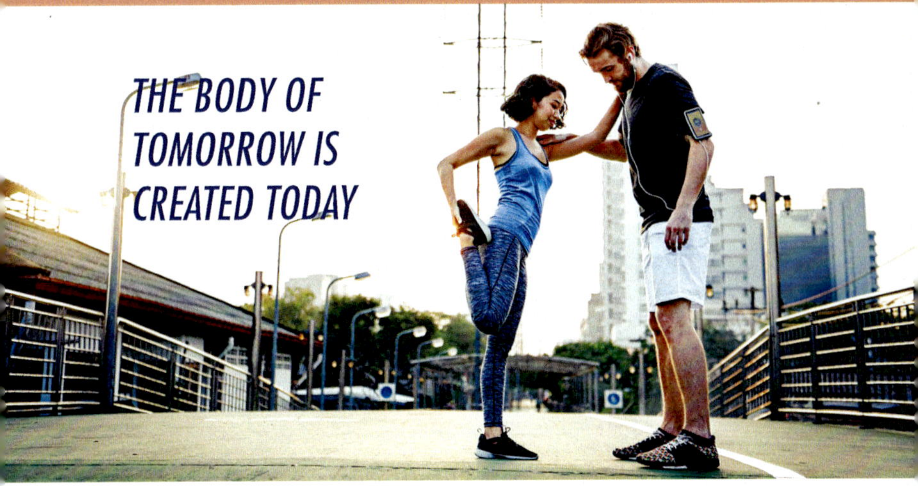

NOTES

5
SUGAR FREE CHALLENGE

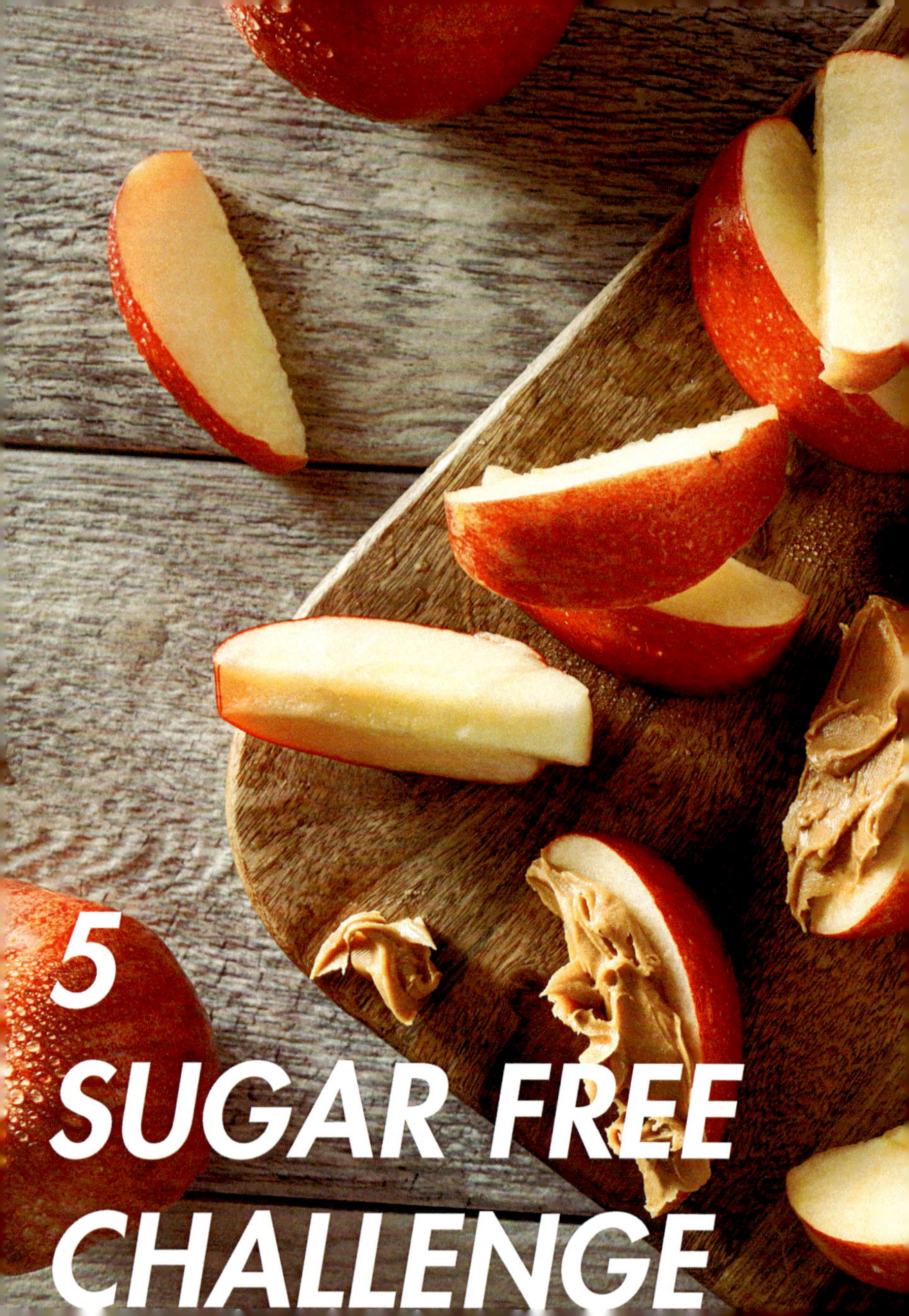

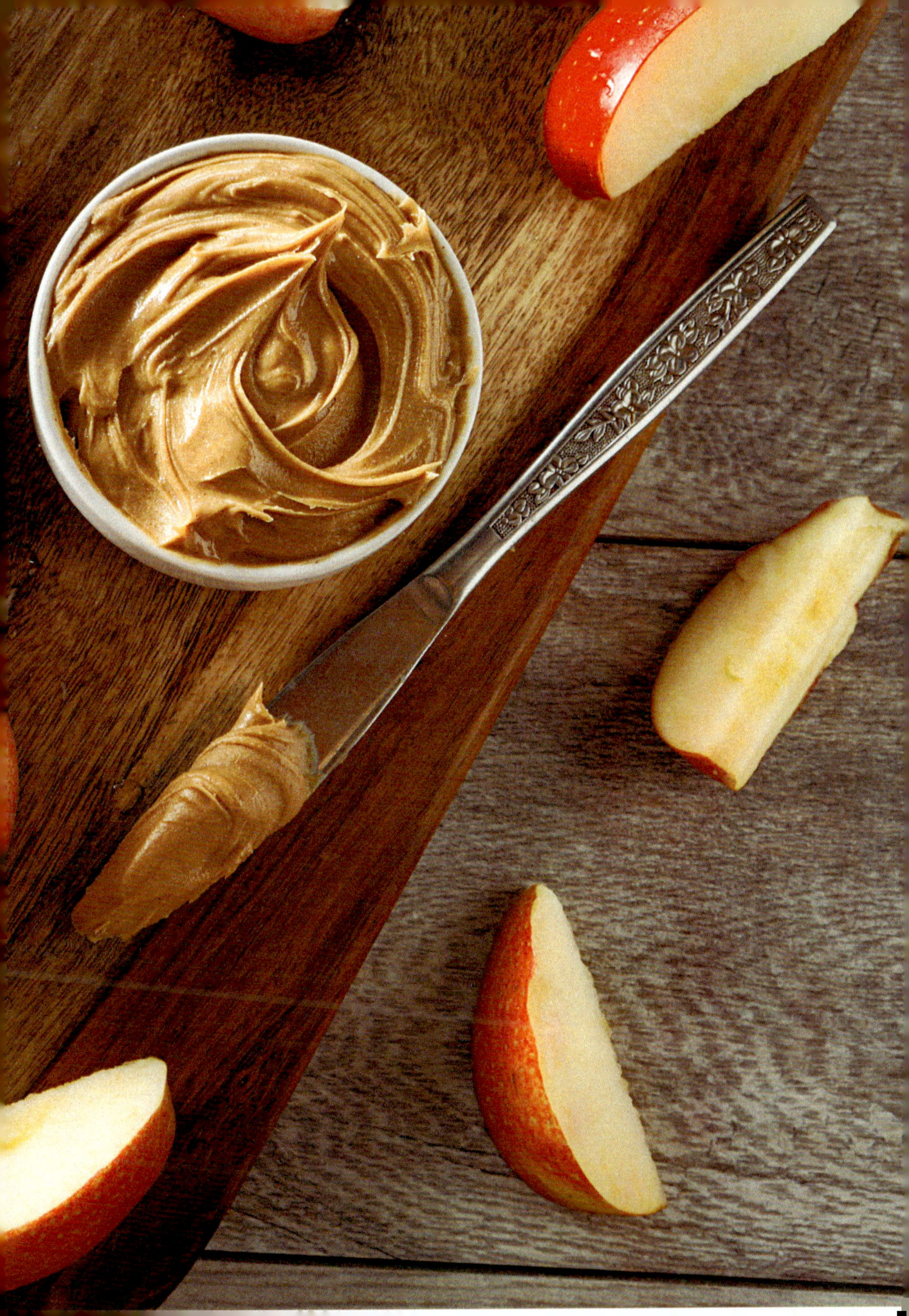

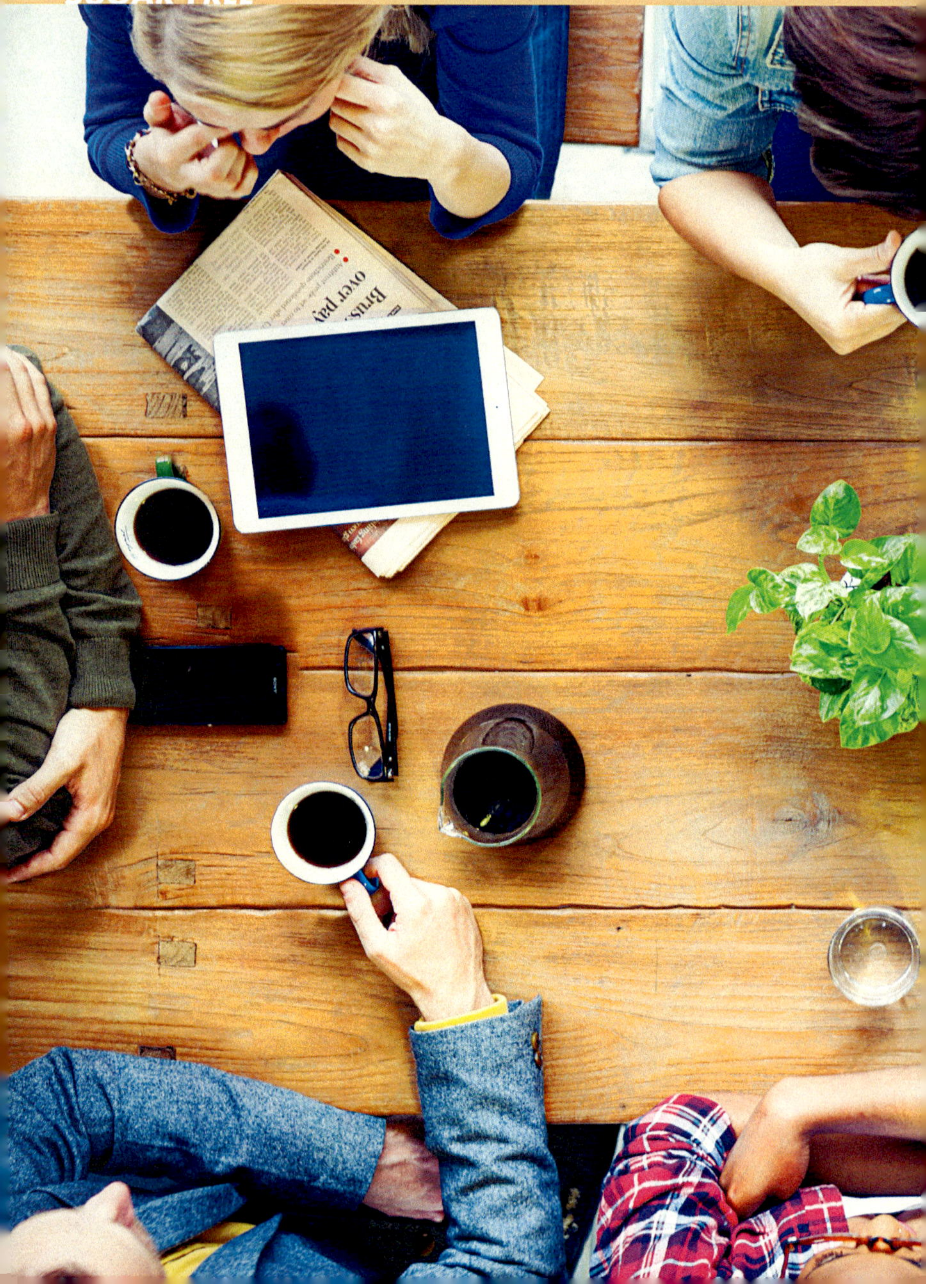
over pay

WHY GO SUGAR FREE?

Sugar is rich in calories, but lacks nutritional value, which is why it's commonly referred to as empty calories. For this reason, sugar added to your food is strongly associated with weight gain and malnutrition. This may seem obvious, but the sources of added sugar may not. [23]

The majority of added sugar comes from processed and prepared foods such as breads, crackers and juice along with the unquestionably sweetened jams, chocolates and ice cream. [24] As a result, many unaware American's consume significant amounts of hidden sugar, which leads to weight gain or obesity.

The second leading cause of preventable disease in America is excess weight or obesity, which increases the risk of many health conditions including the following: [25]

› ***Coronary heart disease, stroke, and high blood pressure***

› ***Type 2 diabetes***

› ***Cancers, such as endometrial, breast, and colon cancer***

› ***High total cholesterol or high levels of triglycerides***

› ***Liver and gallbladder disease***

› ***Sleep apnea and respiratory problems***

› ***Degeneration of cartilage and underlying bone within a joint (osteoarthritis)***

› ***Reproductive health complications such as infertility***

› ***Mental health conditions***

HOW TO SPOT THE SUGAR IN NUTRITION LABELS

The Food and Drug Administration requires labels in order to keep you informed. They do this because corporations are driven by profits, and profits are determined by sales. In order to maximize sales and still stay within the bounds of FDA labeling requirements, alternative names are used to describe sugar.

Here are some alternative names for 'sugar': [26]

Agave nectar
Barley malt
Beet sugar
Brown sugar
Cane juice
Cane sugar
Carob syrup
Coconut palm sugar
Corn syrup
Date sugar
Dehydrated cane juice
Dextrin
Dextrose
Fructose
Fruit juice
Fruit juice concentrate
Glucose
HFCS (High-Fructose Corn Syrup)
Honey
Malt syrup
Maltodextrin
Maltol
Maltose
Mannose
Maple Syrup
Molasses
Palm sugar
Panocha
Powdered sugar
Raw sugar
Rice syrup
Saccharose
Sorghum syrup
Sucrose
Sugar (granulated)
Sweet Sorghum
Syrup
Treacle
Turbinado sugar
Yellow sugar

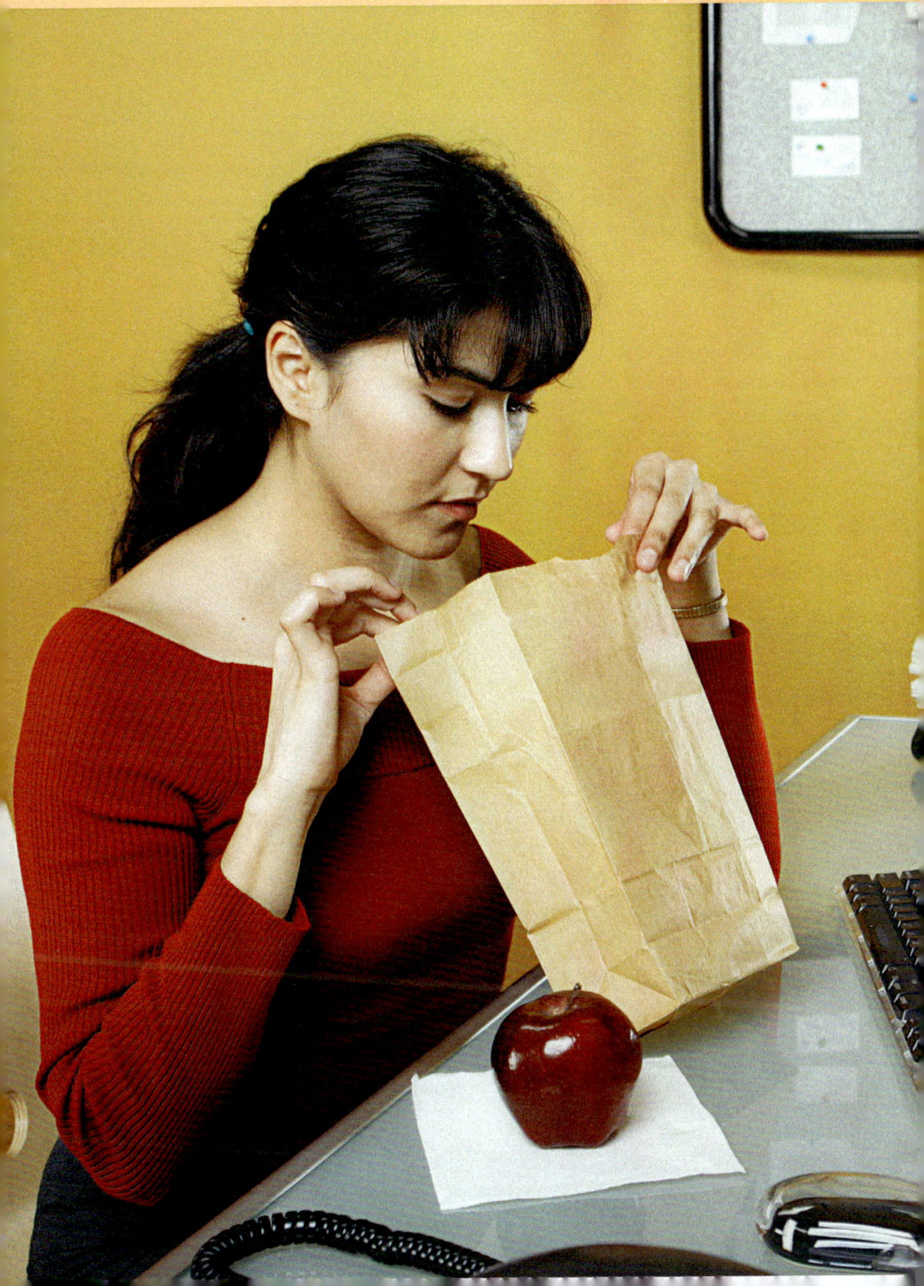

21 DAY SUGAR FREE CHALLENGE

Full Participation involves an elimination of added sugar and sugar alternatives for 21 days. You may consume fruits and vegetables but not in their juiced form. Journal any added sugar or sugar alternatives you consume with each meal.

If this is your first time participating and you feel a complete elimination of sugar and sugar alternatives is beyond your ability, set a goal of consuming 25 or less grams of added sugar but eliminate all sugar alternatives.

(Eat real food and read your labels.)

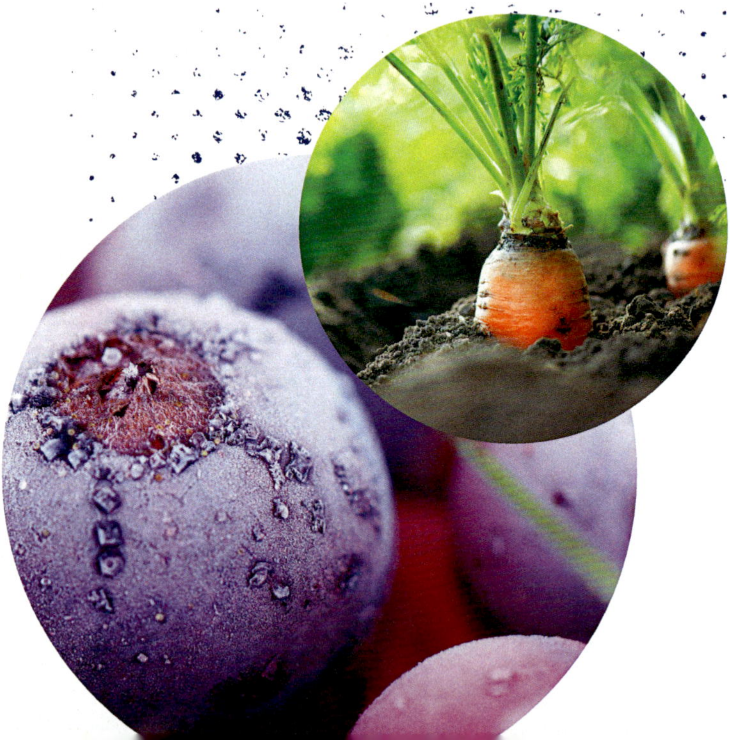

Journal any added sugar or sugar alternatives you consume with each meal, your mood, and hunger levels.

DATE: MOOD ENERGY

MORNING:

I tsp of sugar with coffee

 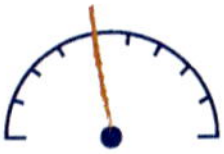

MIDDAY:

none

 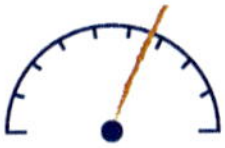

EVENING:

none

 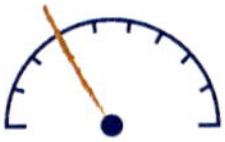

DATE: MOOD ENERGY

MORNING:

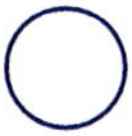 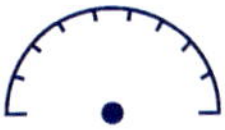

MIDDAY:

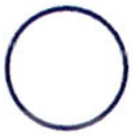 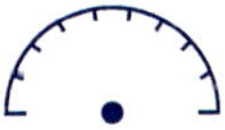

EVENING:

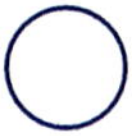 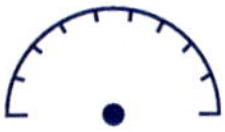

2

DATE: MOOD ENERGY

MORNING:

MIDDAY:

EVENING:

3

DATE: MOOD ENERGY

MORNING:

MIDDAY:

EVENING:

DATE: MOOD ENERGY

MORNING:

MIDDAY:

EVENING:

DATE: MOOD ENERGY

MORNING:

MIDDAY:

EVENING:

6

DATE: MOOD ENERGY

MORNING:

MIDDAY:

EVENING:

7

DATE: MOOD ENERGY

MORNING:

MIDDAY:

EVENING:

DATE: | MOOD | ENERGY

MORNING:

MIDDAY:

8

EVENING:

DATE: | MOOD | ENERGY

MORNING:

MIDDAY:

9

EVENING:

10

DATE: MOOD ENERGY

MORNING:

MIDDAY:

EVENING:

11

DATE: MOOD ENERGY

MORNING:

MIDDAY:

EVENING:

12

DATE: MOOD ENERGY

MORNING:

MIDDAY:

EVENING:

13

DATE: MOOD ENERGY

MORNING:

MIDDAY:

EVENING:

14

DATE: MOOD ENERGY

MORNING:

MIDDAY:

EVENING:

15

DATE: MOOD ENERGY

MORNING:

MIDDAY:

EVENING:

16

DATE: MOOD ENERGY

MORNING:

MIDDAY:

EVENING:

17

DATE: MOOD ENERGY

MORNING:

MIDDAY:

EVENING:

18

DATE: | MOOD | ENERGY

MORNING:

MIDDAY:

EVENING:

19

DATE: | MOOD | ENERGY

MORNING:

MIDDAY:

EVENING:

20

DATE: MOOD ENERGY

MORNING:

MIDDAY:

EVENING:

21

DATE: MOOD ENERGY

MORNING:

MIDDAY:

EVENING:

6 GRATITUDE CHALLENGE

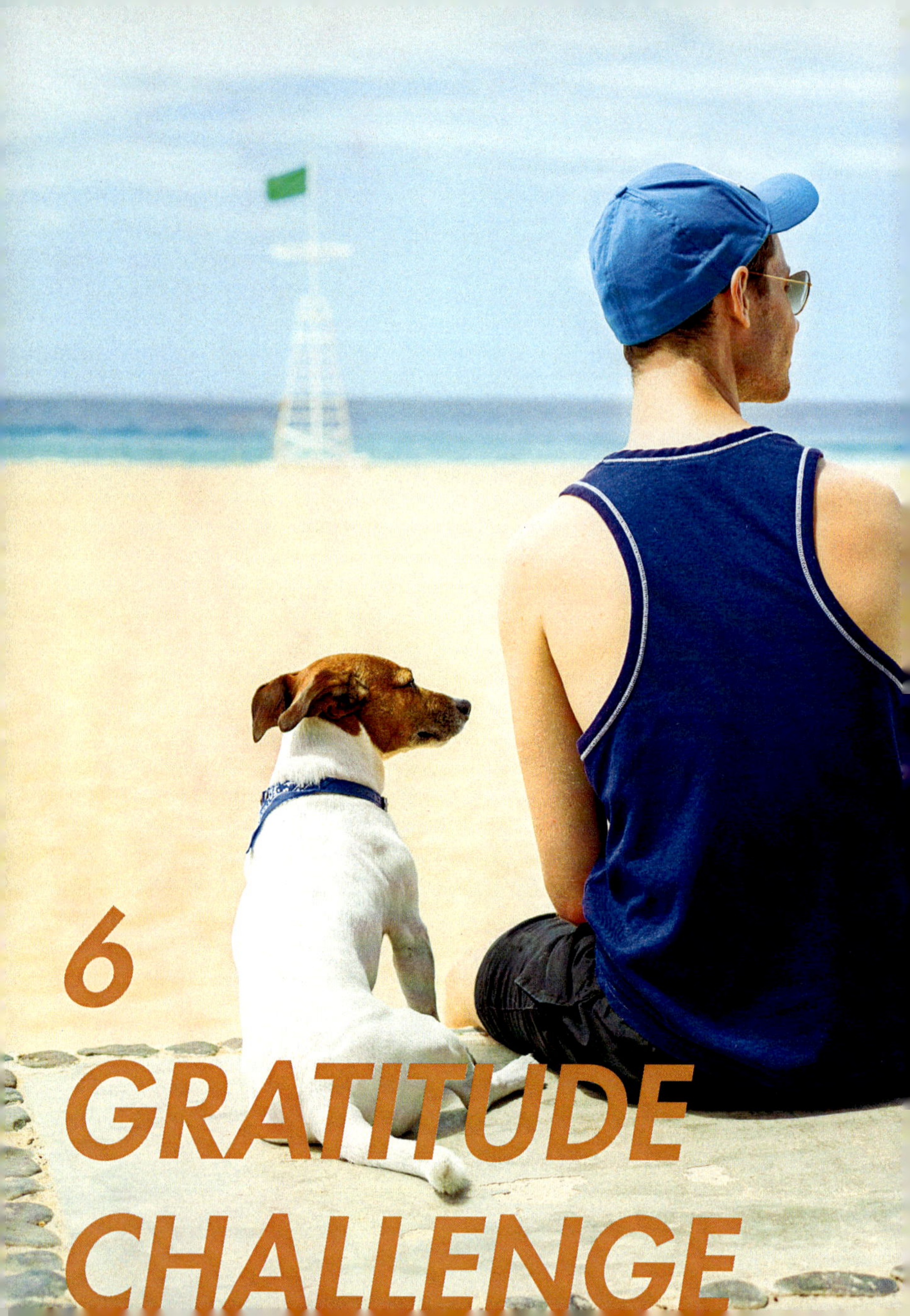

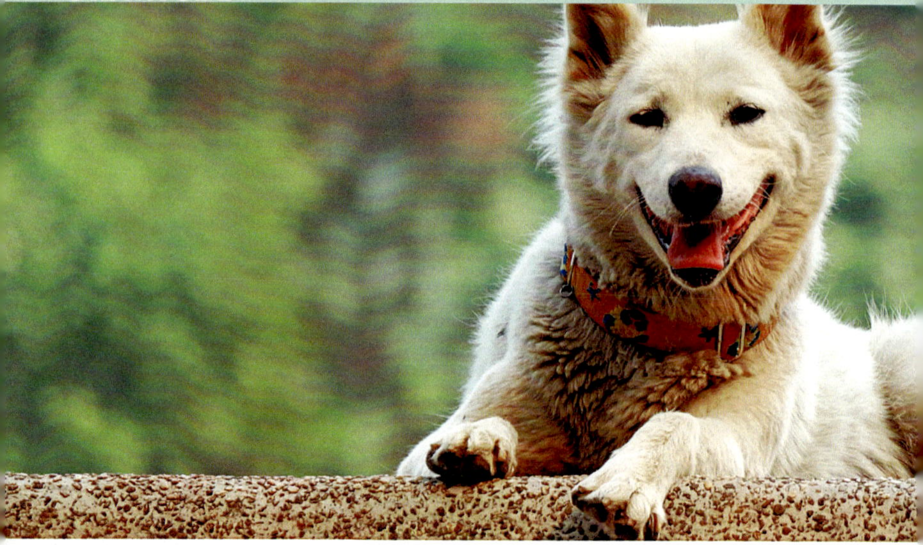

ARE YOU TAKING GRATITUDE FOR GRANTED?

Materially speaking, Americans may have it better than someone in a third world country who earns less than $1000 a year, but having more money doesn't mean we are more satisfied with life. It's estimated 10% of Americans are depressed, 50% of marriages end in divorce, and 70% of Americans hate their job – which explains why there's a tremendous need to look beyond our current circumstances. [27]

Your first step toward a happier and healthier you is to be grateful. Journaling your gratitude for as little as three weeks has been shown to improve physical, psychological and social well-being.

In the research of happiness, gratitude has been shown to be associated with positive emotions, mental alertness, better relationships and improvements in health. [28, 29]

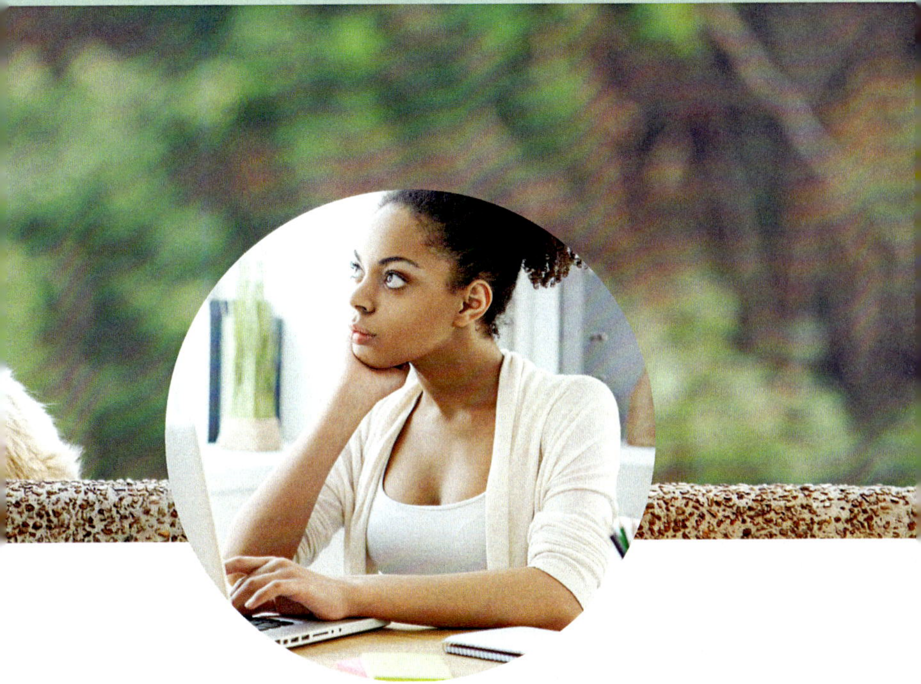

GIVING THANKS LEADS PEOPLE TO:

› *Have stronger immune systems*
› *Express more joy, optimism and happiness*
› *Feel less lonely and isolated*
› *Exercise more regularly*
› *Have improved sleep*
› *Feel more alert, alive and awake*
› *Express more generosity and compassion for others*
› *Be more forgiving of others*

THE 21 DAY GRATITUDE CHALLENGE

› ***Each day, identify one thing for which you are grateful for and a reason why. Journal your results in the First21 Gratitude Challenge Journal.***

› ***Identify a different gratitude each time. Remember the reason WHY you are grateful may be repeated more than once.***

Visit www.first21.com for examples of gratitude

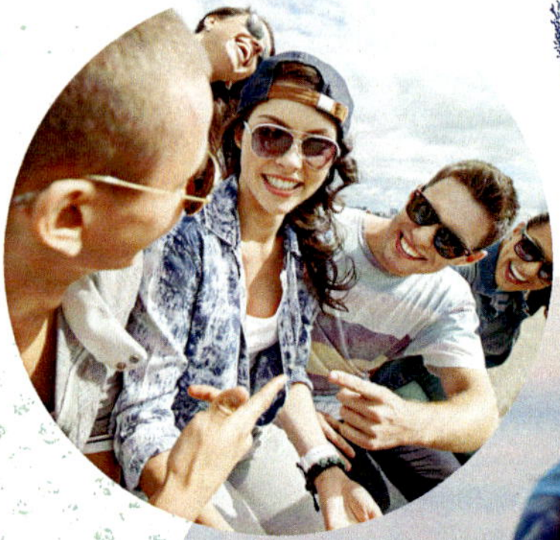

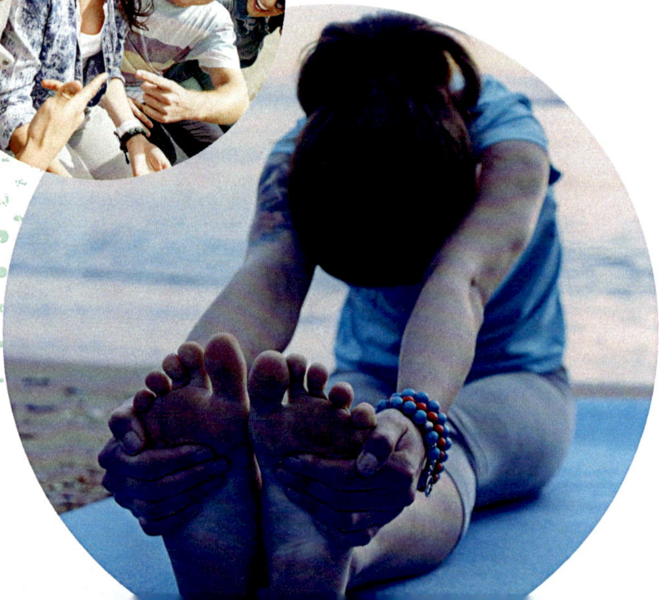

Each day, journal what you are grateful for and why

DATE:

FOR WHAT, AND WHY, ARE YOU GRATEFUL TODAY?

DATE:

FOR WHAT, AND WHY, ARE YOU GRATEFUL TODAY?

DATE:

FOR WHAT, AND WHY, ARE YOU GRATEFUL TODAY?

DATE:

FOR WHAT, AND WHY, ARE YOU GRATEFUL TODAY?

4

DATE:

FOR WHAT, AND WHY, ARE YOU GRATEFUL TODAY?

5

DATE:

FOR WHAT, AND WHY, ARE YOU GRATEFUL TODAY?

6

DATE:

FOR WHAT, AND WHY, ARE YOU GRATEFUL TODAY?

DATE:

FOR WHAT, AND WHY, ARE YOU GRATEFUL TODAY?

DATE:

FOR WHAT, AND WHY, ARE YOU GRATEFUL TODAY?

DATE:

FOR WHAT, AND WHY, ARE YOU GRATEFUL TODAY?

10

DATE:

FOR WHAT, AND WHY, ARE YOU GRATEFUL TODAY?

11

DATE:

FOR WHAT, AND WHY, ARE YOU GRATEFUL TODAY?

12

DATE:

FOR WHAT, AND WHY, ARE YOU GRATEFUL TODAY?

13

DATE:

FOR WHAT, AND WHY, ARE YOU GRATEFUL TODAY?

14

DATE:

FOR WHAT, AND WHY, ARE YOU GRATEFUL TODAY?

15

DATE:

FOR WHAT, AND WHY, ARE YOU GRATEFUL TODAY?

16

DATE:

FOR WHAT, AND WHY, ARE YOU GRATEFUL TODAY?

17

DATE:

FOR WHAT, AND WHY, ARE YOU GRATEFUL TODAY?

18

DATE:

FOR WHAT, AND WHY, ARE YOU GRATEFUL TODAY?

19

DATE:

FOR WHAT, AND WHY, ARE YOU GRATEFUL TODAY?

20

DATE:

FOR WHAT, AND WHY, ARE YOU GRATEFUL TODAY?

21

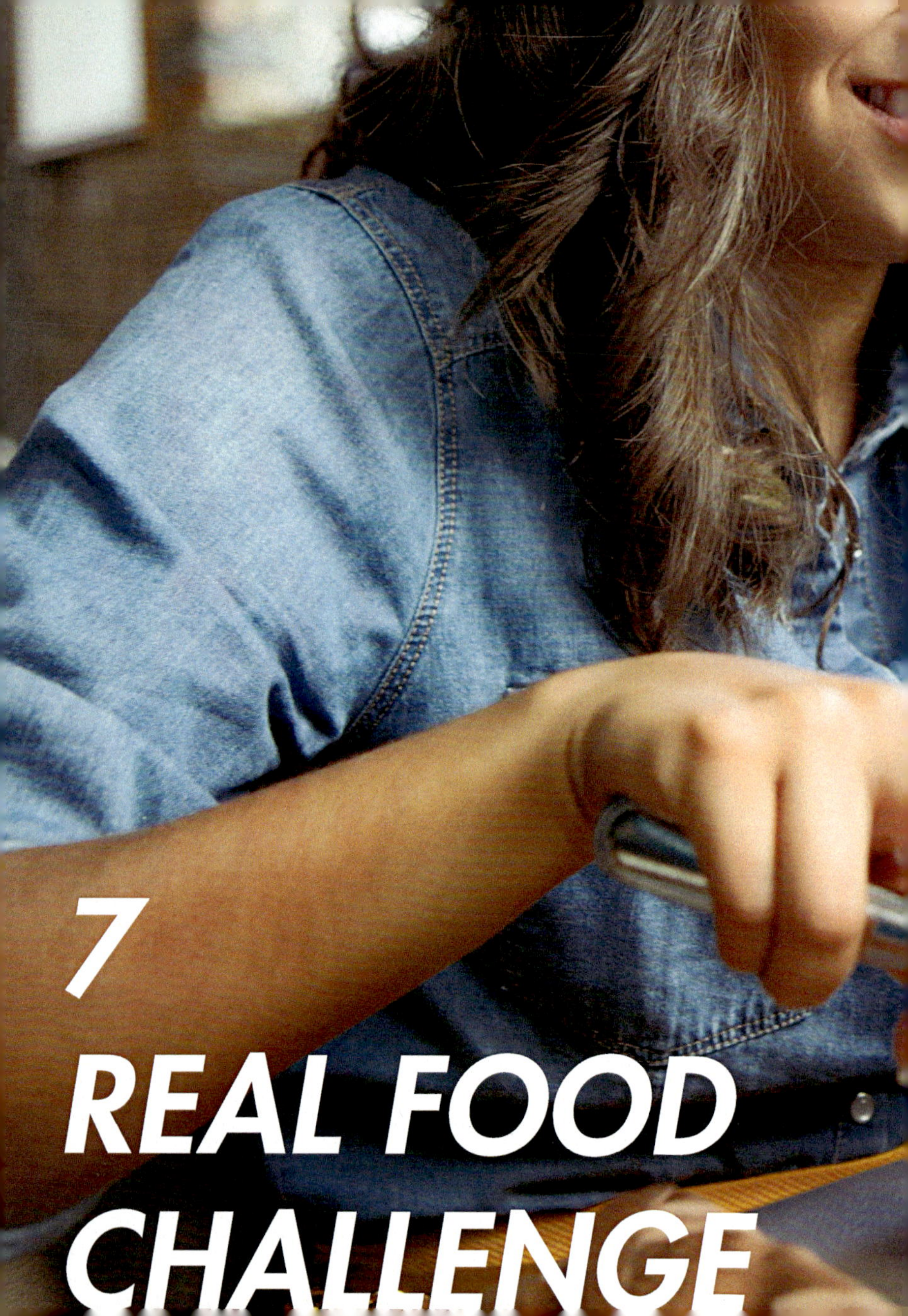

7 REAL FOOD CHALLENGE

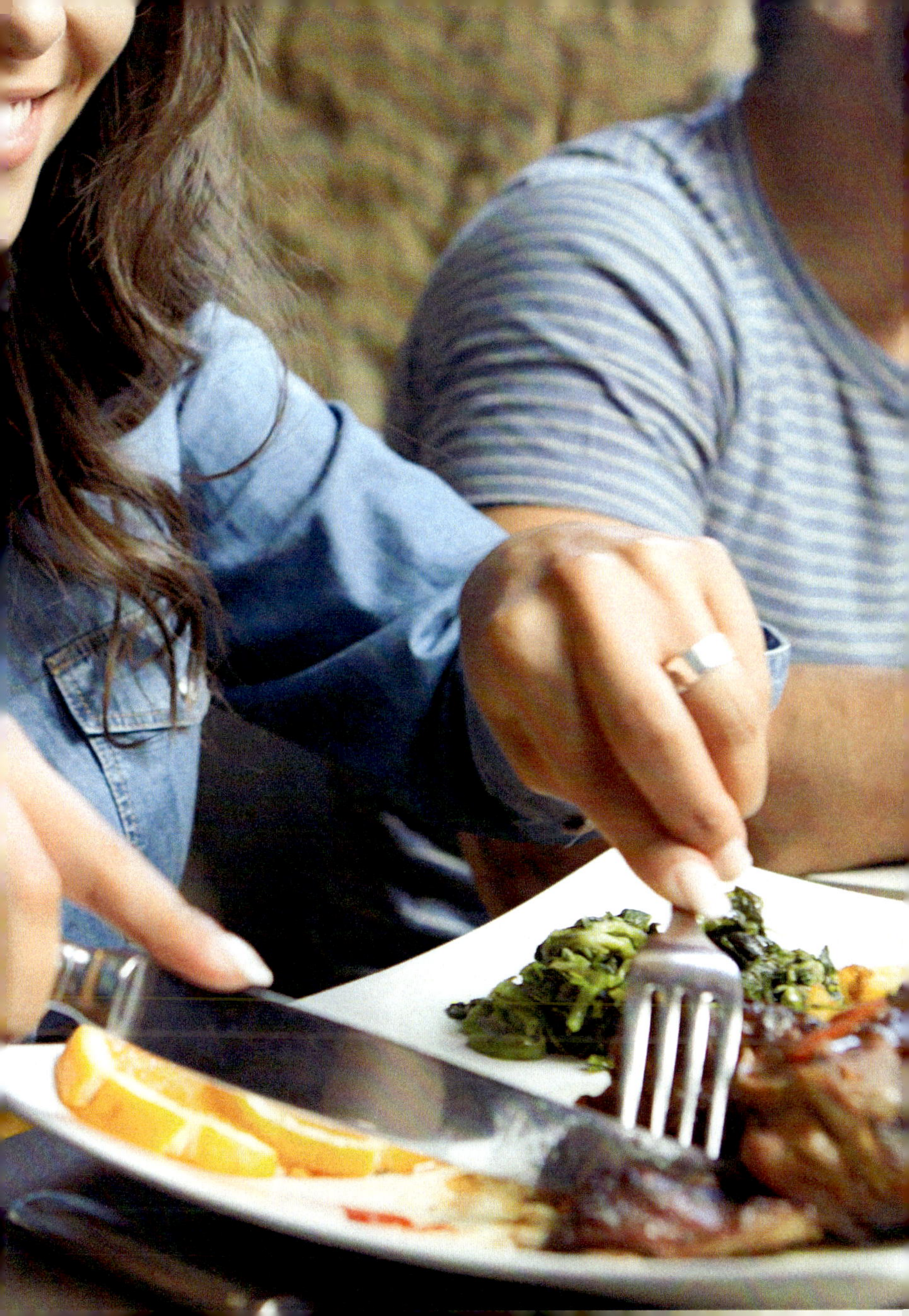

FIRST, LET'S TALK ABOUT THE ALL-AMERICAN DIET

The most common diet consumed in America is called the Standard American Diet (SAD), and it wasn't created by nutritionists. The SAD diet was created by our habits and desires, and supported by large corporations.

It's 'SAD' in lots of ways. This is a diet rich in sugary, processed carbohydrates including cereals, breads, pastas, cookies, candies and cakes. It includes commercially raised and highly processed meat and dairy products, but is almost devoid of grass-fed meat, wild caught fish, vegetables and fruits. [30]

The Real Food Challenge is the most difficult of all the First21 Challenges because it requires you to eliminate added sugars, sugar alternatives and other commonly consumed processed foods and drinks, which might be causing you pain or discomfort.

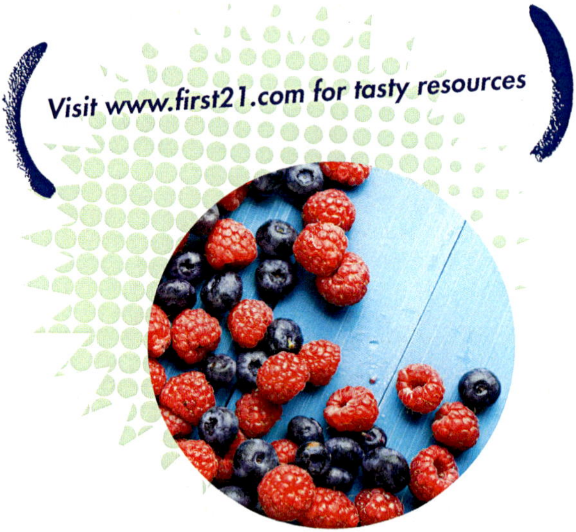

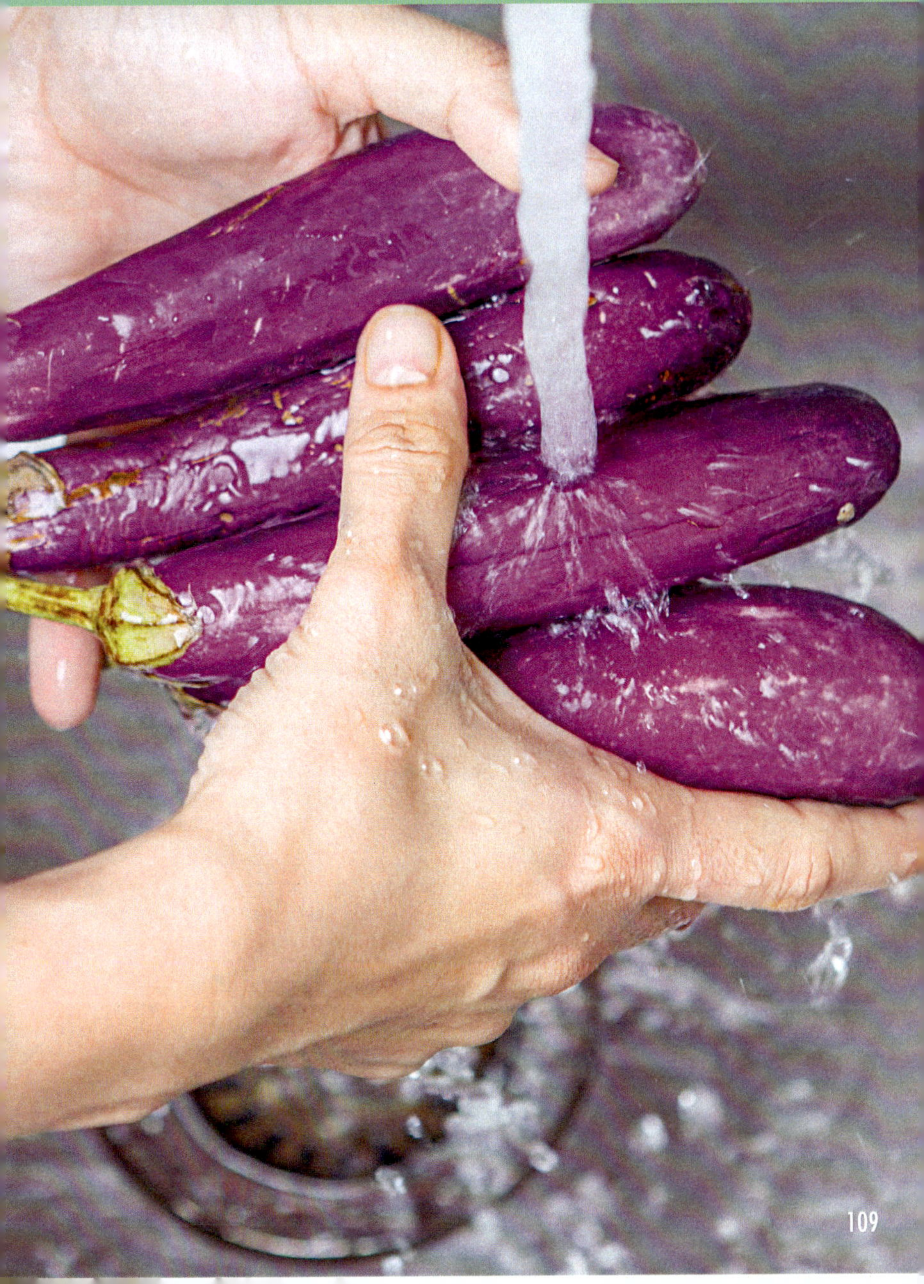

NUTRITION 101

Before you start, it's good to know some basics of nutrition. Nutritionists break down food into three macronutrients called proteins, fats and carbohydrates, all of which are essential in order for your body to function optimally.

Proteins are made up of amino acids, which give your body structure and function, and can be consumed in the form of meat, eggs, milk and beans.

Fats are a source of energy and serve many functions. They insulate your body, help your nerve system run more efficiently, assist in vitamin absorption, and are important for healthy hair and skin. Fats are commonly consumed in the form of fish, seeds, nuts and oils.

Carbohydrate is a complicated word for anything broken down into smaller forms of sugar. Carbohydrates are the primary source of your body's energy, and are either considered simple or complex depending on the amount of sugars in their structure.

– Simple Carbohydrates contain one or two sugars which are rapidly digested because of their simple structure. As a result they can cause rapid spikes in blood sugar levels and be more detrimental than beneficial to your health.. Some of the common sources of simple carbohydrates include cane sugar, brown sugar, corn syrup, honey, molasses & maple syrup. [16, 17] A list of simple sugars is located on page 81.

Simple carbohydrates are also the most common source of "added sugar" in processed foods and may be labeled in their chemical form. Be sure to review the more comprehensive list of sugar names under reading labels for sugar.

– Complex Carbohydrates contain three or more sugars in their structure. They can further be broken down into starchy or non-starchy carbohydrates.

Non-starchy carbohydrates are typically the flowering part of plants and include lettuce, spinach, asparagus, broccoli, cauliflower, cucumber, peppers, tomatoes, zucchini and onions.

Starchy Carbohydrates are higher in their sugar content and commonly consumed in the form of processed grains such as pastas, breads, and rice, or as vegetables as potatoes, yams, pumpkin, and squash. If your goals include weight loss it's important to limit the amount of starchy carbohydrates you consume because of their higher sugar content.

DURING THE REAL FOOD CHALLENGE:

› ***Prepare foods as close as possible to their natural state - the less processed the better***

› ***Ask yourself, "Is this real food or is it food processed in a way to make it appear natural?"***

› ***At the grocery store, stick to the outside isles***

› ***When eating out, order salads with grilled or roasted meat, and ask for vegetables instead of processed pastas and breads, which contain or are quickly converted to sugars***

AFTER THE REAL FOOD CHALLENGE YOU WILL HAVE TWO CHOICES:

› ***You may feel so good that you may want to continue eating this way***

› ***Or, you may want to test the waters by slowly reintroducing these foods***

Feeling bloated, fatigued or sick when reintroducing a particular food is a great indicator your body does not fare well. Remember, it can take weeks, if not longer, for the body to heal from damage created by food and food-like items. The First21 Real Food Challenge is an important step toward your improved health and vitality.

THE REAL FOOD CHALLENGE RULES

Participating in the Real Food Challenge will allow you to reduce dependency on processed foods, sugars and foods found to commonly aggravate the digestive system. A list of foods to avoid are listed below.

For the next 21 days you can enjoy:

Delicious grass-fed meat, wild caught seafood, poultry and eggs. You can eat fresh vegetables and fruits, but try to eat more vegetables than fruit. A good goal to strive toward would be 2 or 3 vegetables for every 1 fruit consumed. Cook with good fats like ghee, coconut oil, olive oil or avocado oils. Eat small amounts of nuts and seeds on your salads, as a snack or mixed in your meals.

Avoid the following during the Real Food Challenge:

Sugar or Sugar Alternatives

No cane sugar, honey, dates, maple syrup, or sugar alternatives such as Splenda, Equal, Nutrasweet, or Stevia. Remember to read your nutrition labels for hidden sugars.

Grains including wheat, rice, corn, oats, rye, barley, millet, bulgur, sorghum, buckwheat, sprouted grains, bran, germ and starch

Gluten is a protein found in many common grains including wheat, rye, barley and more. About 3 million Americans have celiac disease, which is caused by an allergic reaction to gluten. Unfortunately, the majority of people with celiac disease are unaware they have it. Some people may even react poorly to gluten without the full allergic reaction. This condition is called non-celiac gluten sensitivity, which can cause symptoms like bloating, gas, diarrhea, headache, fatigue and joint pain. [33, 34]

Grains also contain phytic acids or phytates and lectins, which are antinutrients. Phytic acids cause problems because they bind to important minerals, which causes poor absorption and potential malnutrition. Lectins protect a plant's reproduction by irritating and therefore stopping the gut from digesting them. Essentially lectins allow you to pass on a plant's seeds to a new location. Lectins have been associated with symptoms including diarrhea, nausea, bloating, reflux and vomiting. [35, 36, 37, 38]

Legumes like black beans, red beans, pinto beans, navy beans, white beans, kidney beans, lima beans, fava beans, chickpeas and lentils

This includes any bean hummus, peanuts, peanut butter, and all forms of soy. Legumes also have lectins (see above under grains for issues associated with lectins).

Dairy including cow's, goat's or sheep's milk and their products, including cream, cheese, yogurt, butter and sour cream.

The first thought for many when considering the elimination of dairy is, "I need dairy's calcium for my bones." But research has shown dairy has no benefit for bone health. In 2005 an article in Pediatrics, the official journal of the American Academy of Pediatrics, milk consumption was shown to not improve bone integrity in children.[39] Even the highly regarded Harvard Nurses' Health Study, which followed 72,000 women for 18 years, showed no protective effect on fracture risk with the consumption of milk. [40]

Even more alarming is the number of people without the natural ability to digest dairy products. Lactose intolerance is a condition where the body doesn't produce enough lactase needed to digest the sugar lactose contained in dairy products. Approximately 95% of Asian-Americans, 74% of Native Americans, 70% of African-Americans, 53% of Mexican Americans and 15% of Caucasian-Americans are considered lactose intolerant. [41]

Artificial flavor enhancers or food preservatives

Eliminate all added Monosodium glutamate (MSG), nitrates, nitrites, sulfites & other preservatives or additives.

Alcohol You're committed to 21 days of clean eating and clear thinking!

EXCEPTIONS TO THE RULES:

Clarified Butter or Ghee

Salted and unsalted butters are not allowed during the challenge, but you may consume clarified butter or ghee. Non-clarified butter contains milk proteins.

Specific Legumes

Green beans, sugar snap peas and similar veggies can be more "pod" than "bean", making them better for you than the alternative legumes.

HERE'S HOW TO HELP YOURSELF:

Use your knowledge and experience from other First21 challenges

By now you've already completed the sugar-free and veggie challenge, so you know your resistance to taking on a new regime. You know your weak spots and vulnerability better than anyone else, but you also know how strong your willpower levels have become. Use the pointers, recipes and strategies you've learned from other challenges to make the Real Food challenge successful.

Schedule the next 21 days in advance.

It's easier to make bad food choices than good ones. Set yourself up for success by writing down your meals in advance. Keeping a consistent meal plan can be one of your best tools while integrating other strategies and pointers. Don't forget to visit www.first21.com for recipe ideas.

Meal Preparation

Pick one or two days to prepare meals for your week. Vacuum seal and freeze meals for a later date. Do anything to make yourself more successful during the First21 real food challenge and beyond.

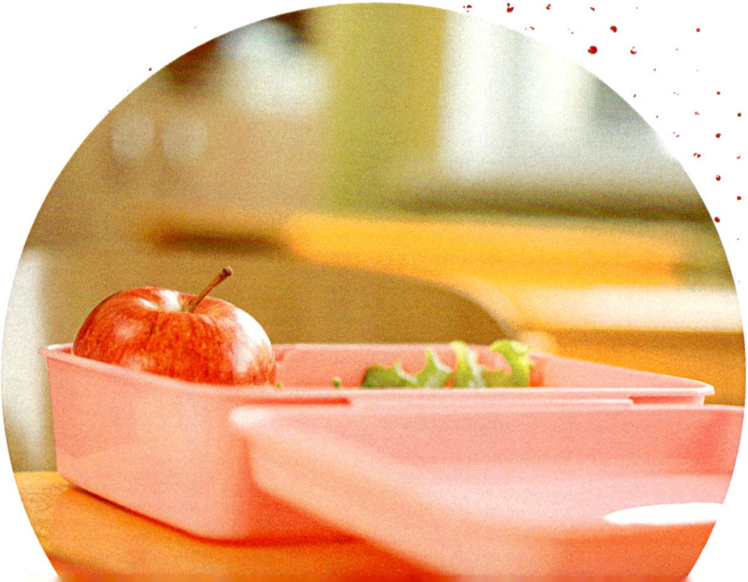

Write down what you eat each day, your mood, and your energy levels.

DATE: 5/23 — MOOD — ENERGY LEVEL

MORNING: egg white omelette
coffee and almond milk
snack: spinach, banana, mango smoothie

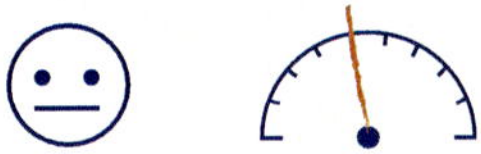

MIDDAY: spinach salad with snap peas,
wasabi dressing, chicken with bbq sauce,
snack: blueberries

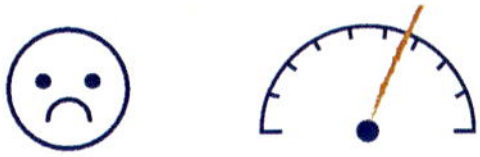

EVENING: salmon, green beans with
stevia and sesame seeds, almond milk

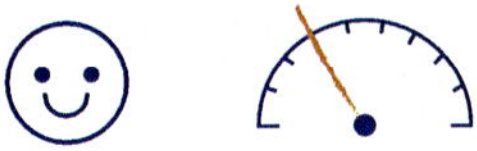

DATE: — MOOD — ENERGY LEVEL

MORNING:

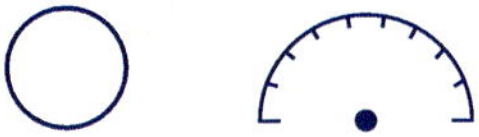

MIDDAY:

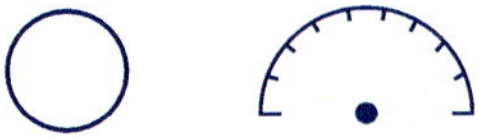

EVENING:

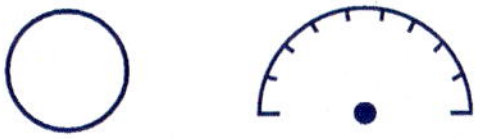

2

DATE: MOOD ENERGY LEVEL

MORNING:

MIDDAY:

EVENING:

3

DATE: MOOD ENERGY LEVEL

MORNING:

MIDDAY:

EVENING:

DATE: MOOD ENERGY LEVEL

MORNING:

MIDDAY:

EVENING:

DATE: MOOD ENERGY LEVEL

MORNING:

MIDDAY:

EVENING:

6

DATE: MOOD ENERGY LEVEL

MORNING:

MIDDAY:

EVENING:

7

DATE: MOOD ENERGY LEVEL

MORNING:

MIDDAY:

EVENING:

8

DATE: MOOD ENERGY LEVEL

MORNING:

MIDDAY:

EVENING:

9

DATE: MOOD ENERGY LEVEL

MORNING:

MIDDAY:

EVENING:

DATE: MOOD ENERGY LEVEL

MORNING:

MIDDAY:

EVENING:

10

DATE: MOOD ENERGY LEVEL

MORNING:

MIDDAY:

EVENING:

11

12

DATE: MOOD ENERGY LEVEL

MORNING:

MIDDAY:

EVENING:

13

DATE: MOOD ENERGY LEVEL

MORNING:

MIDDAY:

EVENING:

DATE: MOOD ENERGY LEVEL

MORNING:

MIDDAY:

14

EVENING:

DATE: MOOD ENERGY LEVEL

MORNING:

MIDDAY:

15

EVENING:

DATE: MOOD ENERGY LEVEL

MORNING:

MIDDAY:

16

EVENING:

DATE: MOOD ENERGY LEVEL

MORNING:

MIDDAY:

17

EVENING:

18

DATE: MOOD ENERGY LEVEL

MORNING:

MIDDAY:

EVENING:

19

DATE: MOOD ENERGY LEVEL

MORNING:

MIDDAY:

EVENING:

DATE: MOOD ENERGY LEVEL

MORNING:

MIDDAY:

20

EVENING:

DATE: MOOD ENERGY LEVEL

MORNING:

MIDDAY:

21

EVENING:

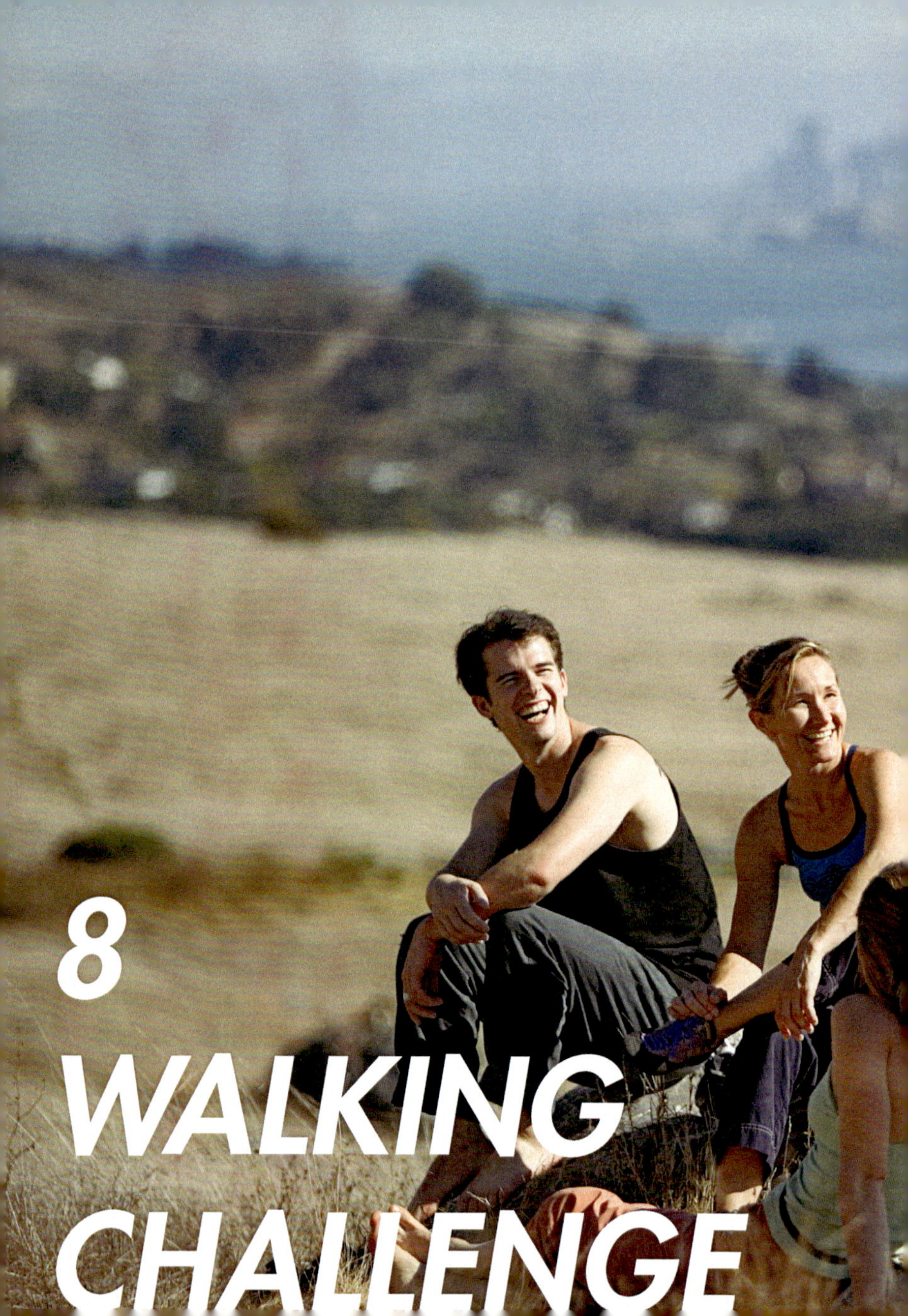

8 WALKING CHALLENGE

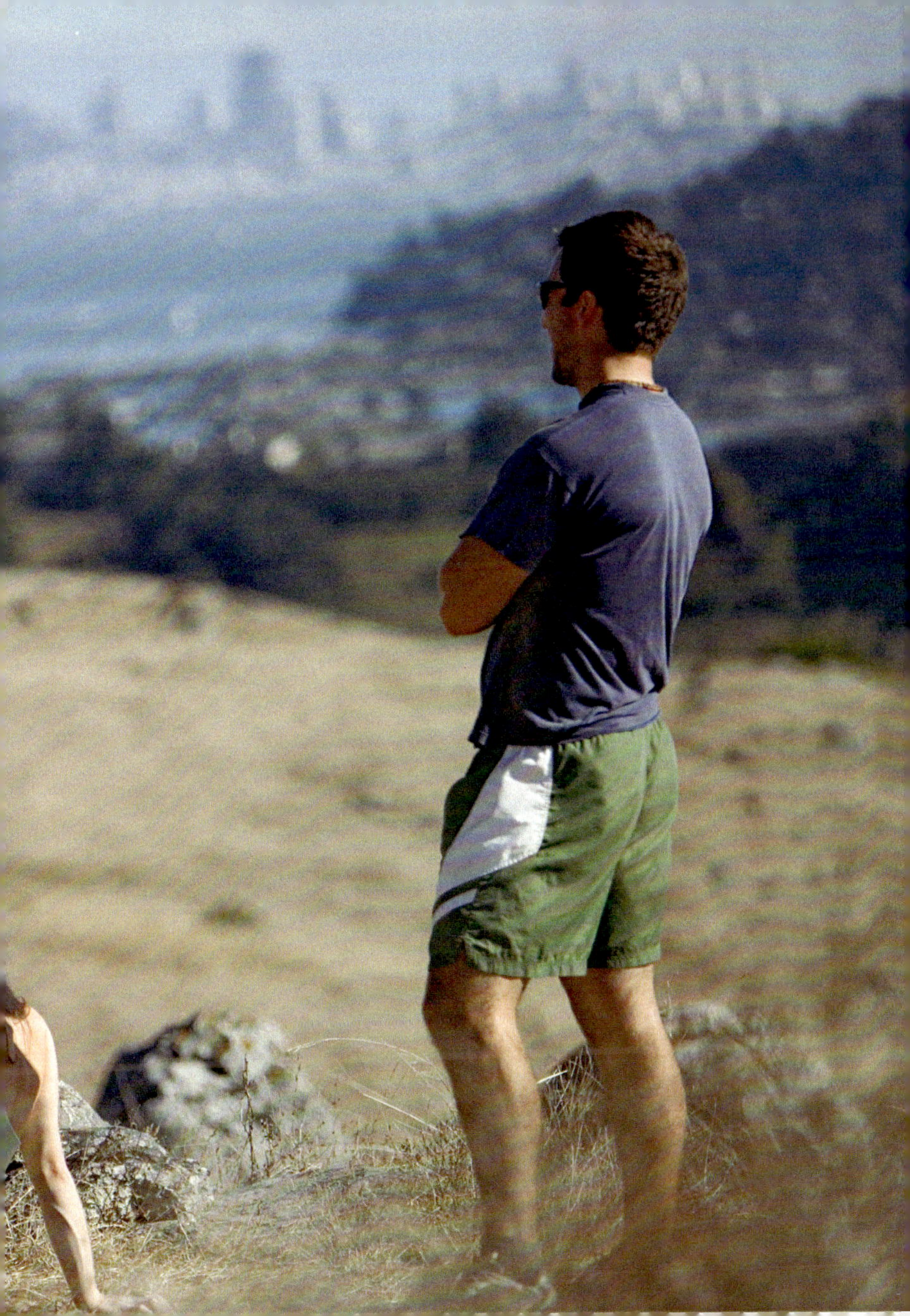

LET'S WALK!

The First21 series of challenges is designed for you to be able to complete and repeat over one year – with one exception. We're giving you a bonus Walking Challenge. Why? Because walking is so easy, and so good for you.

We can all benefit from walking, whether we're super-fit athletes or couch potatoes. It's the ultimate in improving your mind and body at the same time. In fact, we're betting you won't even find your daily walk to be challenging at all.

THE FACTS

According to the Center for Disease Control (CDC) less than half of Americans are exercising enough. CDC stats show only 48% meet the standards of its Physical Activity Guidelines, which recommends adults participate in moderate level physical activity at least 150 minutes a week. [42]

Divide the recommended minutes into seven days and you would only need to exercise a little over 21 minutes a day to meet the CDC's minimum recommendations.

HOW MANY HOURS A DAY DO YOU SIT?

If you are not walking you are most likely sitting; sitting in your car, at a desk, or on the sofa. This is a big problem. In fact, prolonged sitting is associated with obesity, diabetes, heart disease, metabolic syndrome and premature death. [43] It's time to take action, and for many of us this should begin with walking.

When it comes to exercise there isn't a more accessible and easy movement – plus, it's free!

Walking requires spatial awareness, balance, core stability and synchronized movement between the upper and lower body. In addition, walking for at least 30 minutes a day has been shown to reduce the risk of coronary heart disease, osteoporosis, breast and colon cancer, obesity and Type 2 diabetes, and to improve blood sugar and generally make us happier. [44]

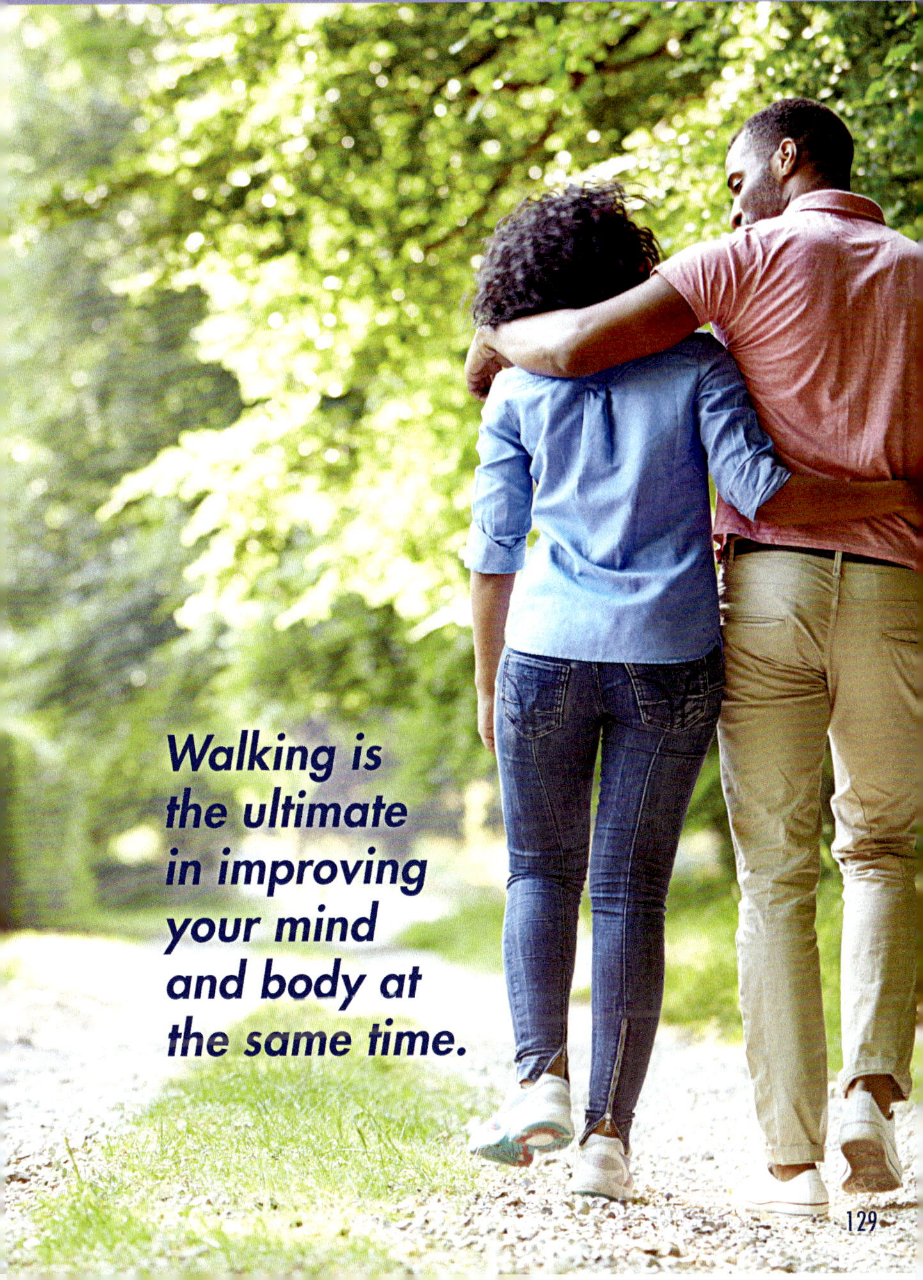
Walking is the ultimate in improving your mind and body at the same time.

HOW TO MAKE WALKING A PART OF YOUR DAY:

Start or end the day with a 5 to 30 minute walk

Take 5 minute walking breaks at work

Start a lunchtime walking group

Walk your kids to school

Watch your favorite shows while walking on a treadmill

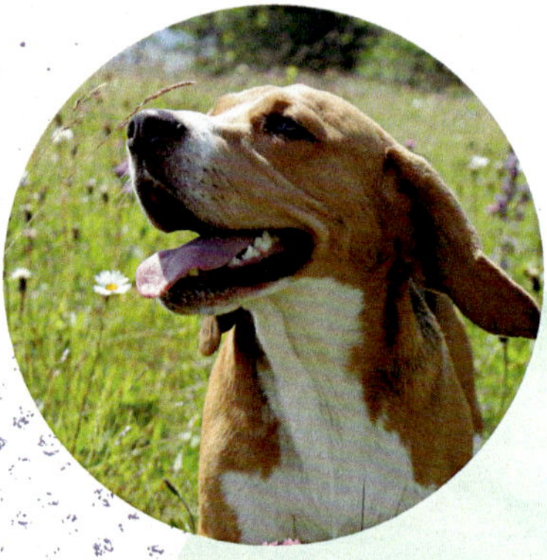

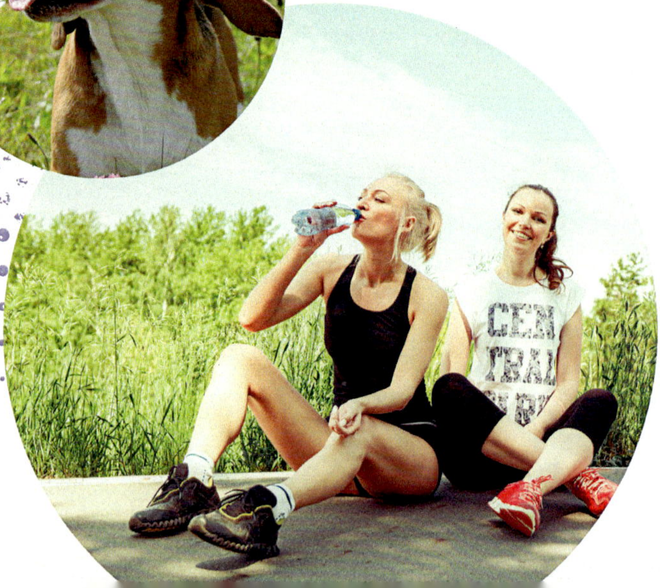

LISTEN TO YOUR BODY

Injuries are more common if you ignore your body's signals of fatigue, discomfort, tightness and pain.

› *Visit your doctor for a full medical check-up before starting any exercise program*

› *Respect your current fitness level by starting an exercise program at a pace you can maintain*

› *Injuries require rest and recovery. Working through pain will only cause more damage and delay healing*

› *If you have a pre-existing injury or are prone to injury, consult your doctor before starting this exercise program*

STOP EXERCISING AND SEEK MEDICAL HELP IF YOU EXPERIENCE ANY OF THE FOLLOWING SYMPTOMS:

› *Pain or discomfort*

› *Chest pain that could indicate a heart attack, including pain in the neck, jaw, pain traveling down the arm or pain between the shoulder blades*

› *Breathlessness or inability to catch your breath*

› *Rapid or irregular heartbeat during exercise*

› *Joint pain persisting after more than three days of rest*

FIRST21 WALKING CHALLENGE

Walk 30 minutes each day for 21 days. The 30 minutes of walking can be broken into 5 minute increments as long as it is intentional exercise. As an example, walking as you shop at the grocery store would not count, but intentionally walking the outskirts of the mall, or around the block, or over your lunch break would count.

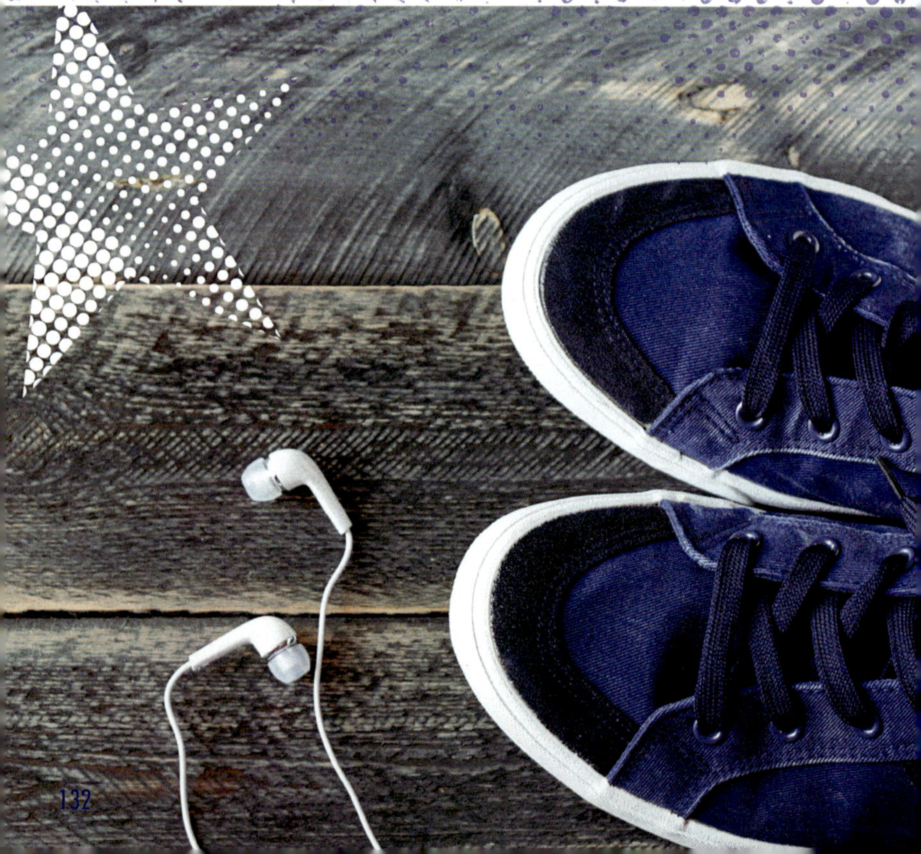

Each day, journal the minutes walked, mood, and energy level.

SAMPLE

DATE: 7/19 | MOOD | ENERGY LEVEL

MORNING: 10 minutes in neighborhood

MIDDAY: 20 min outside office

EVENING: walk dog 30 min

DATE: | MOOD | ENERGY LEVEL

MORNING:

MIDDAY:

EVENING:

DATE: MOOD ENERGY LEVEL

MORNING:

2

MIDDAY:

EVENING:

DATE: MOOD ENERGY LEVEL

MORNING:

3

MIDDAY:

EVENING:

DATE: MOOD ENERGY LEVEL

MORNING:

MIDDAY:

4

EVENING:

DATE: MOOD ENERGY LEVEL

MORNING:

MIDDAY:

5

EVENING:

6

DATE: MOOD ENERGY LEVEL

MORNING:

MIDDAY:

EVENING:

7

DATE: MOOD ENERGY LEVEL

MORNING:

MIDDAY:

EVENING:

8

DATE: MOOD ENERGY LEVEL

MORNING:

MIDDAY:

EVENING:

9

DATE: MOOD ENERGY LEVEL

MORNING:

MIDDAY:

EVENING:

10

DATE: MOOD ENERGY LEVEL

MORNING:

MIDDAY:

EVENING:

11

DATE: MOOD ENERGY LEVEL

MORNING:

MIDDAY:

EVENING:

12

DATE: MOOD ENERGY LEVEL

MORNING:

MIDDAY:

EVENING:

13

DATE: MOOD ENERGY LEVEL

MORNING:

MIDDAY:

EVENING:

14

DATE: MOOD ENERGY LEVEL

MORNING:

MIDDAY:

EVENING:

15

DATE: MOOD ENERGY LEVEL

MORNING:

MIDDAY:

EVENING:

16

DATE: MOOD ENERGY LEVEL

MORNING:

MIDDAY:

EVENING:

17

DATE: MOOD ENERGY LEVEL

MORNING:

MIDDAY:

EVENING:

18

DATE: MOOD ENERGY LEVEL

MORNING:

MIDDAY:

EVENING:

19

DATE: MOOD ENERGY LEVEL

MORNING:

MIDDAY:

EVENING:

20

DATE: MOOD ENERGY LEVEL

MORNING:

MIDDAY:

EVENING:

21

DATE: MOOD ENERGY LEVEL

MORNING:

MIDDAY:

EVENING:

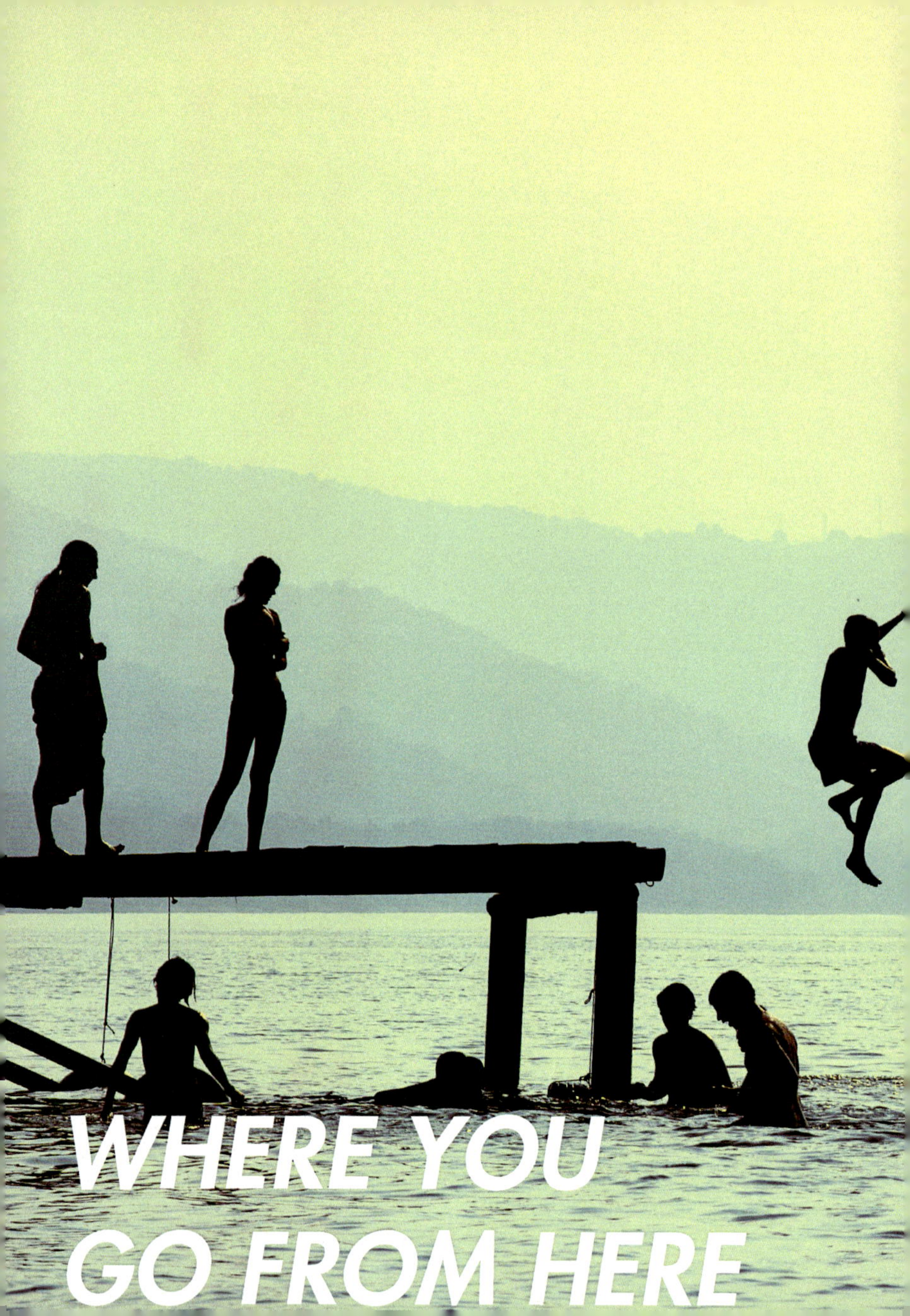

WHERE YOU GO FROM HERE

Maintaining Healthy Habits and Timeless Challenges

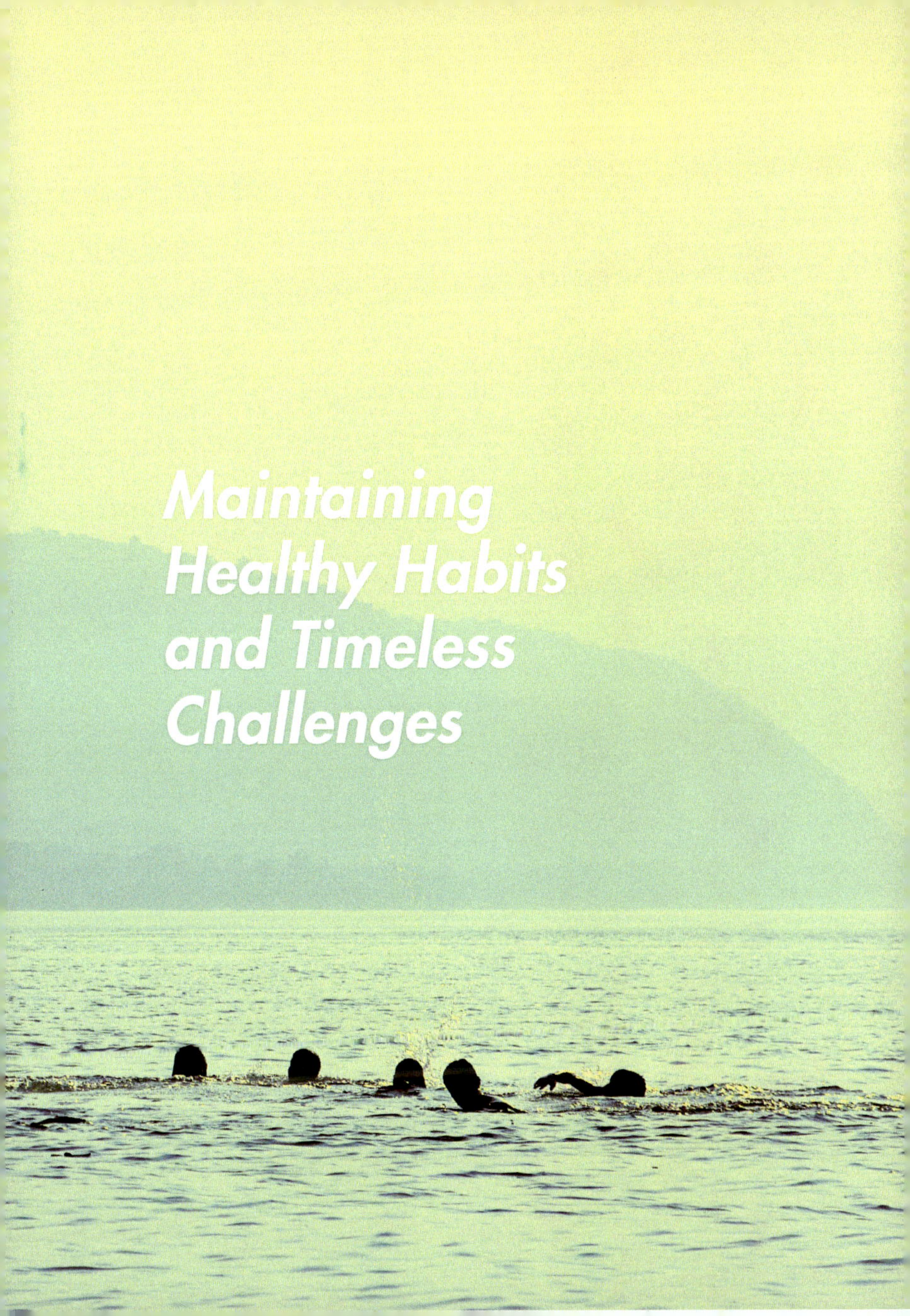

TO REMAIN GOOD AT THIS, YOU NEED TO STICK WITH IT.

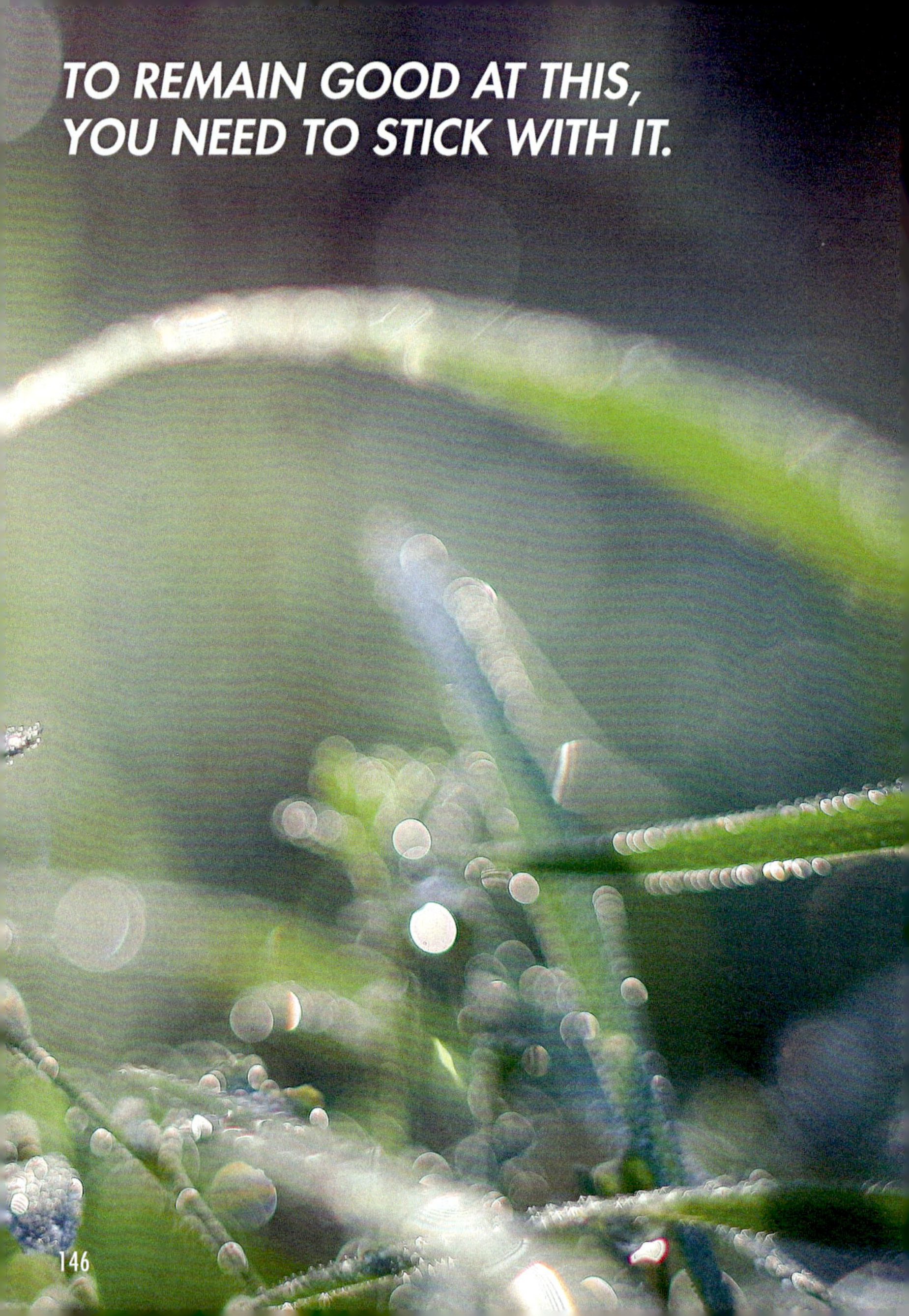

WHAT NOW?

Good question! You've either completed all the First21 Challenges, or you're cheating and skipping to the end of the book. We hope it's the first, and you have successfully completed this program!

But this isn't the end, nor should it be. After mastering the First21 Challenges, you need to repeat them again and again. Remember, we don't intend for this program to be a fad or a passing trend. This is all about you developing new habits for life. It's about re-setting your mind and your body to a healthier way of eating, thinking and moving – timeless healthy habits.

And being good at something – including leading a healthy life – doesn't come without constant practice.

Hopefully you've enjoyed all of the First21 challenges with little to no overwhelm or setbacks. Even if it was a difficult journey, your continued participation will be the key to your success. Repeating these challenges will give you an opportunity to improve, maintain, or even get back on track. This is true even if it's your 100th time through the First21 Challenge.

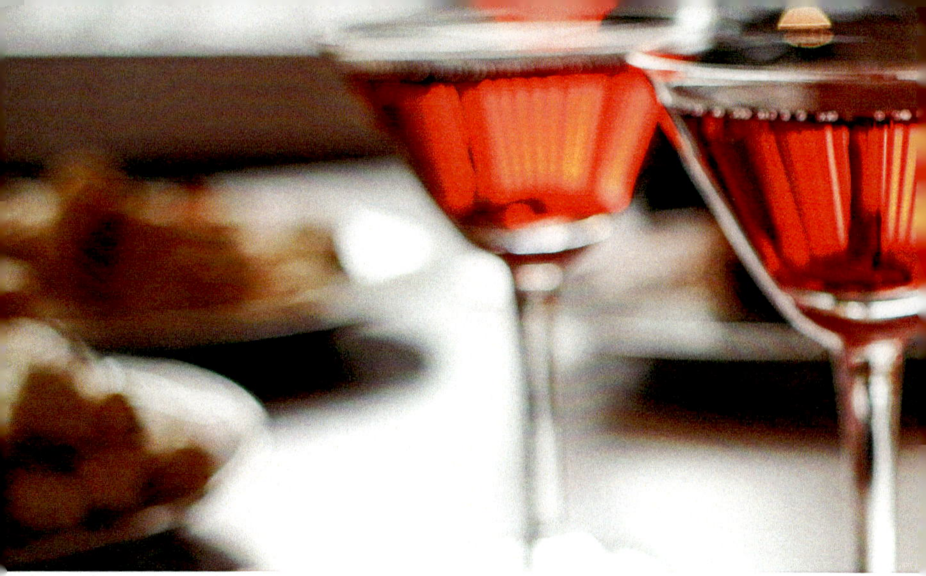

THE BALANCING ACT

For many people, if it has to be all or nothing, they will do nothing. These facts are clearly outlined in the First21 introduction, so we should all be as realistic as we are idealistic. I crave chocolate cake, vanilla bean ice cream, and sometimes enjoy the coma-like nap which follows. Of course, this is not a daily habit, but I'm not always going to deny myself birthday cake and ice cream when given the option.

Remember, the First21 wasn't created to be an all or nothing health program. The goal isn't to participate for 21 days and then go back to your previous ways. Instead, the First21 is an opportunity to incorporate and develop healthy habits which will last a lifetime.

I have read several diet books and blogs suggesting you eat 80/20. This means 80 percent of your choices are healthy allowing for 20 percent to come from the less healthy variety. I have even referenced my own diet as being 80 or 90 percent. This can be useful as a reflection but seems to be a vague recommendation. Additionally, it could lead to a troublesome outcome.

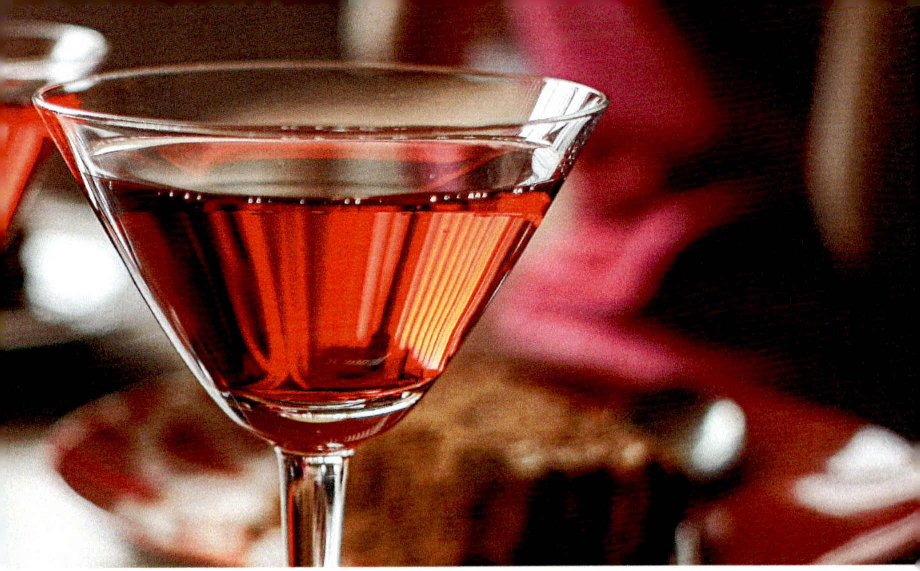

Using the 80/20 rule by the day, week or year would allow you to choose to eat poorly, be inactive and emotionally resentful 73 days per year. Would you want to be around someone unruly 73 days per year? Even worse, would you want to be this person?

Instead of trying to control every variable by a percentage, wouldn't it make more sense to simplify the complexity of wellness and focus on one of many challenging areas each month? This would give you an opportunity to improve or maintain your health every month without the overwhelming goal of perfection.

If you ate way too much sugar last month because of socials, celebrations and holidays, wouldn't it make sense to get back on track with the Sugar Free Challenge? Or, maybe it's the summer and you're planning to travel. Could you bring a stainless steel bottle and participate in the Water Challenge?

My experience with participants has been they make better overall choices as long as they are participating in one of the First21 Challenges each month. In other words, once you complete a challenge, you will keep this challenge at the forefront of your mind even when you are working on a completely different area of your wellness. Awareness is key. When you are aware of your choices, you are more likely to make healthy choices.

BUT WHAT IF...?

What if you fall at the first hurdle? What if you fall after a week? Life is not straightforward, which is why we've posed some questions you might be asking, and some answers to help.

Q: I'm finding it difficult to kick my sweet tooth, even after successfully doing the sugar challenge. Is it OK to stick with artificially sweetened drinks and foods?

A: Occasional sugar isn't the problem. So, enjoy your sugary treat if it's only every once in a while. But, if you need something to take the edge off until you've gotten the no sugar habit down, start with stevia. It's extracted from the leaves of a plant called Stevia rebaudiana, which has been grown for centuries in South America. It's popular because of its natural source, sweet taste and low- to no-calorie effect. My concerns with artificial sweeteners align with many critics who are concerned they may cause a variety of health problems, including cancer. Remember, like athletes who practice to improve performance, you may need to do the Sugar Free Challenge several times before you control your cravings!

Q: I travel a lot, and I find it hard to maintain my new First21 fitness regime. Any tips?

A: What's great about body weight exercises is how they can be done at the gym, at home or even in a hotel room. Prepare yourself for success by scheduling your hotel workouts and be sure to bring necessary clothing.

Q: I have a family wedding coming up right in the middle of my First21 challenge. Help! How can I continue First21 without looking like I'm a fussy eater?

A: Remember, participation is more important than perfection. Eat as healthy as you can and enjoy it without guilt. Journal your "cheats" and then start the next meal or day as if it never happened. In the end you will probably feel guiltier for not eating the meal provided than you will for cheating.

Q: I stay on track with the Challenges until about Day 4, then I fall off the wagon and find it really hard to get back on again. Is there something wrong with me?

A: Sometimes you need to do some prep work before you jump into a challenge. Next time, do the challenge with a small group of your friends for added accountability. Or, schedule everything out a week or more at a time. Things in your schedule are more likely to get accomplished!

Q: I love the new habits I have formed through First21 and now I would like to get my whole family on board. Do you have any advice for bringing reluctant spouses and young children onto the program?

A: Families are tough because they rarely take you as seriously as they would a doctor. The First21 can always become fun by rewarding participants or by turning each challenge into a competition. Whatever you do, be sure to educate the family on "why" to participate and "how" they can benefit from each challenge. Health isn't always the solution to getting someone to participate. Sometimes they need to know they will perform better at a sport or hobby from added strength from exercise. Or, they may think more clearly at work or school from eating less processed foods. The First21 is a balanced program because the challenges are centered on how to improve the way you eat, move and think. There is something for everyone in the First21!

Q: Can I do all the challenges at the same time?

A: If you want to complete all of the challenges simultaneously, go for it! Be sure to journal your successes and enjoy your journey.

I HOPE YOU LIKE THE NEW YOU

You've worked hard to develop your healthy new habits, and you deserve to take a moment to celebrate your achievements – not to mention your clean new mind and body.

When maintaining your First21 habits and your commitment to eating, moving and thinking healthily, it's good to remind yourself why you did this in the first place - and what makes First21 unique and successful. Make them your mantras. Say them to yourself every day. Write them down, carry them with you – whatever it takes:

› ***Health isn't a perfect number on the scale. It's a state of complete physical, mental and social well-being***

› ***Quick-fix diets and fitness regimes simply don't work. You need short-term results to become a long-term solution***

› ***It takes 21 days to break a habit and 21 days to create a new one. Stick with our program for 21 days and you're on the path to a new you***

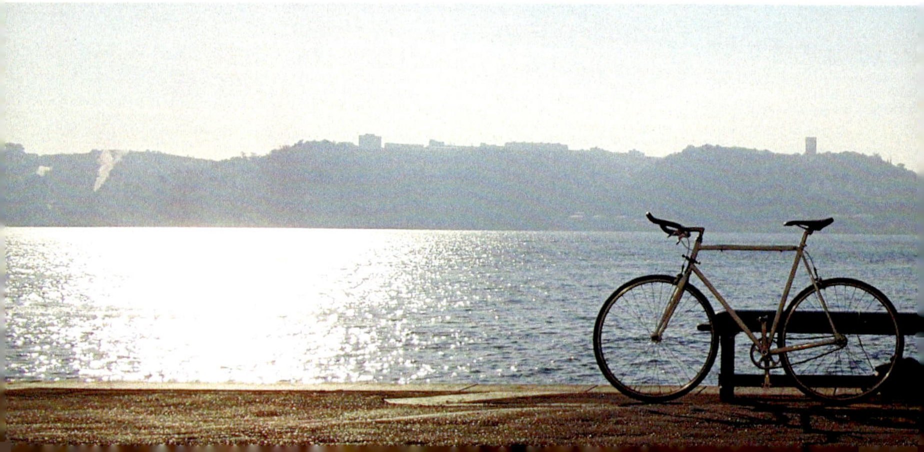

› ***Be grateful. It's the first step to a healthier, happier you***

› ***Eat more vegetables, drink more water, cut out sugar, eat real food***

› ***No time for exercise? No problem. The Tabata challenge only requires a few minutes a day***

I thank you for letting me join you in your journey. And remember, for continuous, updated tips and advice, visit the First21 website at www.first21.com

- Geoff Huls DC, CCWP

FIRST 21

Eat Move Think

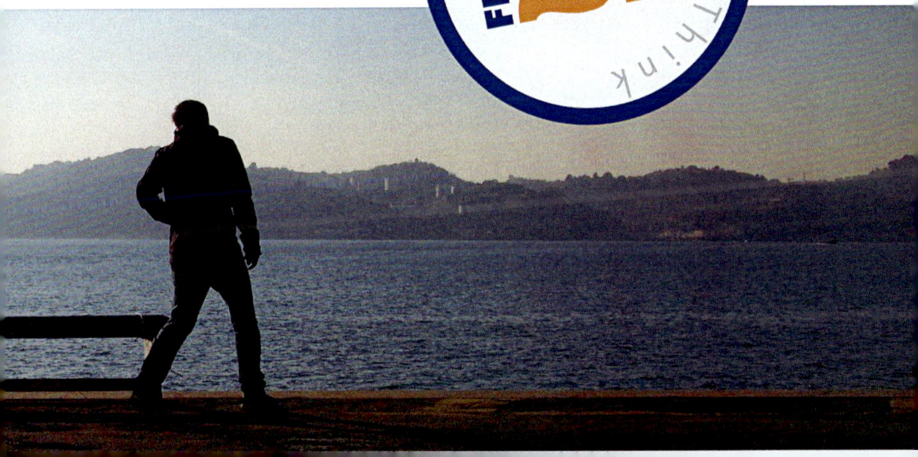

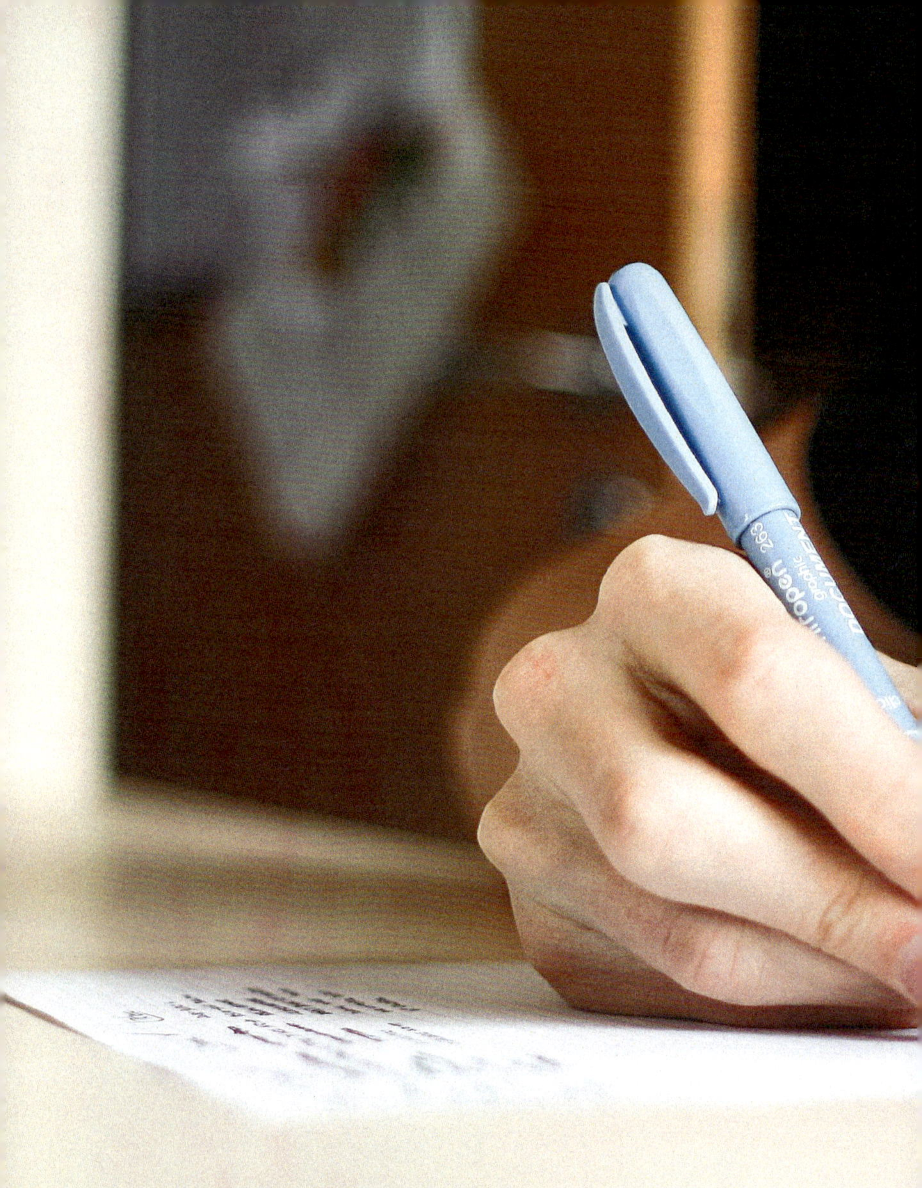

SCHEDULE

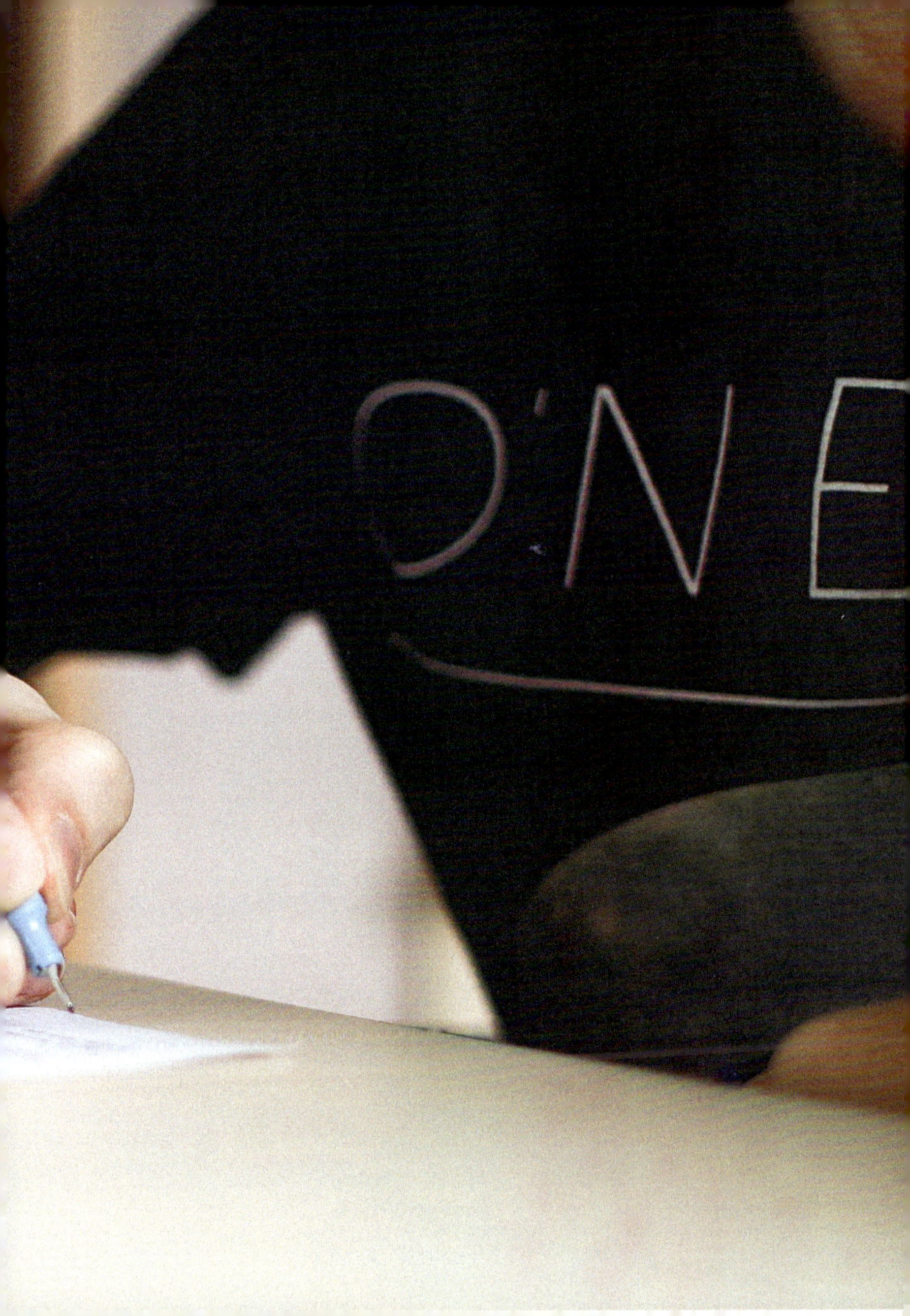
O'NE

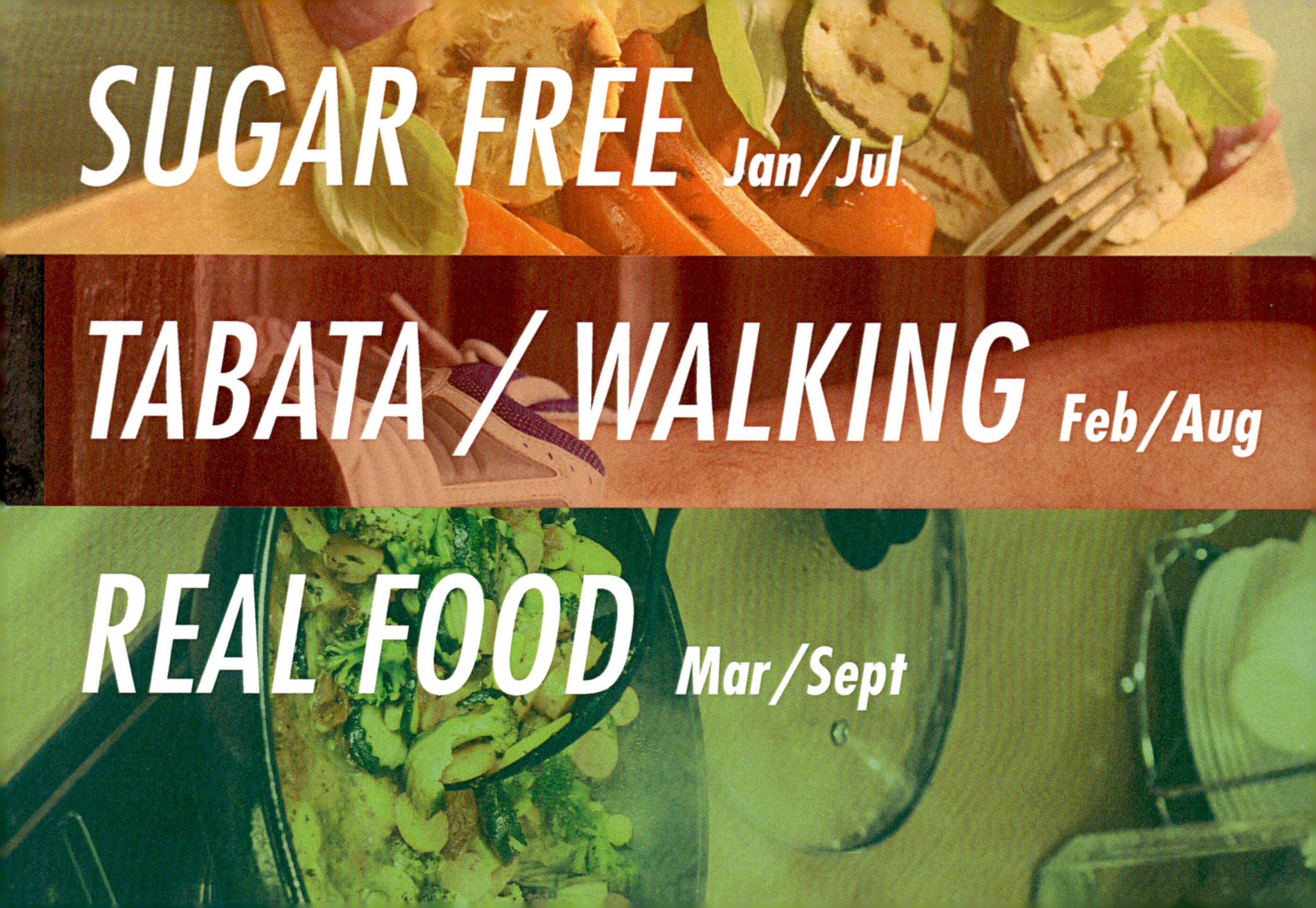
SUGAR FREE Jan/Jul
TABATA / WALKING Feb/Aug
REAL FOOD Mar/Sept

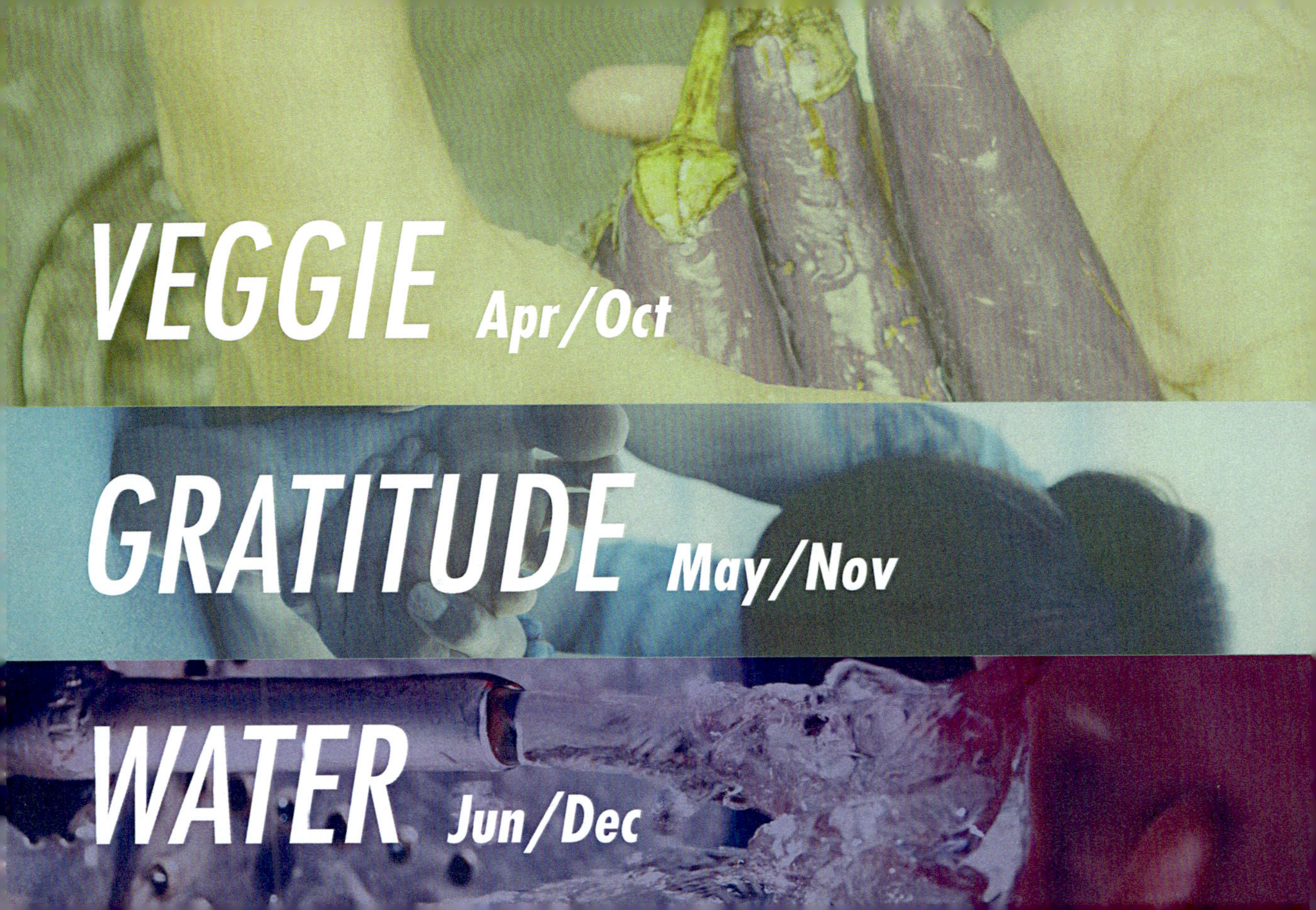
VEGGIE Apr/Oct
GRATITUDE May/Nov
WATER Jun/Dec

END NOTES & BIBLIOGRAPHY

INTRODUCTION

1. Finkelstein E, PhD, MHA; Khavjou O, MA; ThompsonH, BA; Trogdon J, PhD; Liping P, MD, MPH; SherryB, PhD, RD; Dietz W, MD, PhD. "Obesity and SevereObsesity Forecasts Through 2030," American Journal of Preventive Medicine, Volume 42, Issue 6.

2. "Adult Obesity Causes & Consequences." Centers for Disease Control and Prevention. Centers for Disease Control and Prevention, 16 June 2015. Web. 10 July 2016. https://www.cdc.gov/obesity/adult/causes.html

3. Thomas, Thom, Nancy Haase, Wayne Rosamond, Virginia Howard, John Rumsfeld, Teri Manolio, Zhi-Jie Zheng, Katherine Flegal, Christopher O'Donnell, Steven Kittner, Donald Lloyd-Jones, David Goff, Jr., and Yuling Hong. "Heart and Stroke Association Statistics." Heart and Stroke Association Statistics. American Heart Association, 14 Feb. 2006. Web. 14 July 2016. <http://circ.ahajournals.org/content/circulationaha/113/6/e85.full.pdf>.

4. "Family Cancer Syndromes." Family Cancer Syndromes. American Cancer Society, 25 June 2014. Web. 10 July 2016. http://www.cancer.org/cancer/cancercauses/geneticsandcancer/heredity-and-cancer

5. Heyn, H., F. J. Carmona, A. Gomez, H. J. Ferreira, J. T. Bell, S. Sayols, K. Ward, O. A. Stefansson, S. Moran, J. Sandoval, J. E. Eyfjord, T. D. Spector, and M. Esteller. "DNA Methylation Profiling in Breast Cancer Discordant Identical Twins Identifies DOK7 as Novel Epigenetic Biomarker." Carcinogenesis 34.1 (2012): 102-108.

FIRST 21 FOUNDATIONAL CONCEPTS

6. Rhodes DG, Adler ME, Clemens JC, LaComb RP, Moshfegh AJ. "Consumption of Pizza: What We Eat in America," NHANES 2007-2010. Food Surveys Research Group Dietary Data Brief No. 11. February 2014.

VEGGIE CHALLENGE

7. "Tomatoes and Potatoes Are the Most Commonly Consumed Vegetables." United States Department of Agriculture. Economic Research Service., 4 Nov. 2013. Web. 8 July 2016. <http://www.ers.usda.gov/data-products/chart-gallery/detail.aspx?chartId=40452>

8. "Dietary Guidelines." Center for Nutrition Policy and Promotion. USDA, n.d. Web. 10 July 2016. <http://www.cnpp.usda.gov/dietary-guidelines>.

9. Wang, X., Y. Ouyang, J. Liu, M. Zhu, G. Zhao, W. Bao, and F. B. Hu. "Fruit and Vegetable Consumption and Mortality from All Causes, Cardiovascular Disease, and Cancer: Systematic Review and Dose-response Meta-analysis of Prospective Cohort Studies." BMJ 349.Jul 29 3 (2014):349

10. Zhang, X., X.-O. Shu, Y.-B. Xiang, G. Yang, H. Li, J. Gao, H. Cai, Y.-T. Gao, and W. Zheng. "Cruciferous Vegetable Consumption Is Associated with a Reduced Risk of Total and Cardiovascular Disease Mortality." American Journal of Clinical Nutrition 94.1 (2011): 240-246.

11. Williams, David J., David Edwards, Ingrid Hamernig, Le Jian, Anthony P. James, Stuart K. Johnson, and Linda C. Tapsell. "Vegetables Containing Phytochemicals with Potential Anti-obesity Properties: A Review." Food Research International 52.1 (2013): 323-333.

12. He, K., F. B. Hu, G. A. Colditz, J. E. Manson, W. C. Willett, and S. Liu. "Changes in Intake of Fruits and Vegetables in Relation to Risk of Obesity and Weight Gain among Middle-aged Women." International journal of obesity and related metabolic disorders. International Journal of Obesity 28.12 (2004): 1569-1574.

13. Bazzano L. A., T Y Li, K J Joshipura, and F B Hu. "Intake of Fruit, Vegetables, and Fruit Juices and Risk of Diabetes in Women." Diabetes Care 31.7 (2008): 1311-1317

14. Ford, Earl S., and Ali H. Mokdad. "Fruit and Vegetable Consumption and Diabetes Mellitus Incidence among U.S. Adults." Preventive Medicine32.1 (2001): 33-39.

15. John, Jh, S. Ziebland, P. Yudkin, Ls Roe, and Haw Neil. "Effects of Fruit and Vegetable Consumption on Plasma Antioxidant Concentrations and Blood Pressure: A Randomised Controlled Trial." The Lancet 359. 9322 (2002): 1969-1974.

16. "Adults Meeting Fruit and Vegetable Intake Recommendations — United States, 2013." Centers for Disease Control and Prevention. Centers for Disease Control and Prevention, 10 July 2015. Web. 11 July 2016. <http://www.cdc.gov/MMWR/preview/mmwrhtml/mm6426a1.htm>.

WATER CHALLENGE

17. "Water and Nutrition." Centers for Disease Control and Prevention. Centers for Disease Control and Prevention, 03 June 2014. Web. 11 July 2016. <http://www.cdc.gov/healthywater/drinking/nutrition/index.html>.

18. Munoz, Colleen X., Evan C. Johnson, Amy L. Mckenzie, Isabelle Guelinckx, Gitte Graverholt, Douglas J. Casa, Carl M. Maresh, and Lawrence E. Armstrong. "Habbitual Total Water intake and Dimensions of Mood in Healthy Young Women." Appetite 92 (2015): 81-86.

19. Pross, Nathalie, Agnès Demazières, Nicolas Girard, Romain Barnouin, Déborah Metzger, Alexis Klein, Erica Perrier, and Isabelle Guelinckx. "Effects of Changes in Water Intake on Mood of High and Low Drinkers."PLoS ONE 9.4 (2014)

20. Ganio, Matthew S., Lawrence E. Armstrong, Douglas J. Casa, Brendon P. Mcdermott, Elaine C. Lee, Linda M. Yamamoto, Stefania Marzano, Rebecca M. Lopez, Liliana Jimenez, Laurent Le Bellego, Emmanuel Chevillotte, and Harris R. Lieberman. "Mild Dehydration Impairs Cognitive Performance and Mood of Men." British Journal of Nutrition Br J Nutr106.10 (2011): 1535-1543.

21. "Dehydration." Symptoms., 12 Feb. 2014. Web. 08 July 2016. http://www.webmd.com/a-to-z-guides/dehydration-adults

TABATA CHALLENGE

22. TABATA, I. et al. (1996) Effects of moderateintensity endurance and high-intensity intermittent training on anaerobic capacity and VO2 max. MedScience Sports Exercise., 28 (10), p. 1327-1330.

SUGAR FREE CHALLENGE

23. Bethene, Ervin R., and Cynthia L. Ogden. "Consumption of Added Sugars Among U.S. Adults, 2005–2010." NCHS Data Brief, Number 122, May 2013: Web. 11 July 2016. <http://www.cdc.gov/nchs/data/databriefs/db122.pdf

24. Consumption of Added Sugars Among U.S. Adults, 2005–2010. (2013, May 1). Mokdad AH, Marks JS, Stroup DF, Gerberding JL (March 2004).

25. Actual causes of death in the United States, 2000". JAMA 291 (10): 1238–45. doi:10.1001/ jama.291.10.1238. PMID 15010446.

26. "Hidden in Plain Sight." SugarScience.org. N.p., 17 Nov. 2013. Web. 11 July 2016. <http://www.sugarscience.org/hidden-in-plain-sight/>.

GRATITUDE CHALLENGE

27. Adkins, Amy. "Majority of U.S. Employees Not Engaged Despite Gains in 2014." Gallup.com., 28 Jan. 2015. Web. 08 July 2016.

28. Froh, J. J., Bono, G., & Emmons, R. A. (2010). Being grateful is beyond good manners: Gratitude and motivation to contribute to society among early adolescents. Motivation and Emotion Volume 34, 144-157.

29. Emmons, Robert A., and Michael E. Mccullough. "Counting Blessings versus Burdens: An Experimental Investigation of Gratitude and Subjective Well-being in Daily Life." Journal of Personality and Social Psychology 84.2 (2003): 377-89.

REAL FOOD CHALLENGE

30. Grotto, D., and E. Zied. "The Standard American Diet and Its Relationship to the Health Status of Americans." Nutrition in Clinical Practice 25.6 (2010): 603-612.

31. Englyst KN, Englyst HN. Carbohydrate bioavailability. British Journal of Nutrition. 2005;94(1):1-11.

32. Varki A. Biological roles of oligosaccharides: all of the theories are correct. Glycobiology. 1993;3(2):97-130.

33. Gao, Ying, Sigurdur Y. Kristinsson, Lynn R. Goldin, Magnus Björkholm, Neil E. Caporaso, and Ola Landgren. "Increased Risk for Non-Hodgkin Lymphoma in Individuals With Celiac Disease and a Potential Familial Association."Gastroenterology 136.1 (2009): 91-98.

34. Ciacci, Carolina, Luigi Maiuri, Nicola Caporaso, Cristina Bucci, Luigi Del Giudice, Domenica Rita Massardo, Paola Pontieri, Natale Di Fonzo, Scott R. Bean, Brian Ioerger, and Marco Londei. "Celiac Disease: In Vitro and in Vivo Safety and Palatability of Wheat-free Sorghum Food Products." Clinical Nutrition 26.6 (2007): 799-805.

35. "Living With Phytic Acid - Weston A Price." Weston A Price. Weston A Price Foundation, 26 March 2010. Web. 11 July 2016. <http://www.westonaprice.org/health-topics/living-with-phytic-acid/>.

36. Hurrell, Richard F. "Journal of Nutrition." Influence of Vegetable Protein Sources on Trace Element and Mineral Bioavailability. Journal of Nutrition, 1 Sept. 2003. Web. 12 July 2016. <http://jn.nutrition.org/content/133/9/2973S.long>.

37. Cordain, L. "Cereal Grains: Humanity's Double-Edged Sword." Evolutionary Aspects of Nutrition and Health World Review of Nutrition and Dietetics (1999): 19-73.

38. Cordain, Loren, L. Toohey, M. J. Smith, and M. S. Hickey. "Modulation of Immune Function by Dietary Lectins in Rheumatoid Arthritis." British Journal of Nutrition. 83.03 (2000): 207-17.

39. Lanou AJ, Berkow SE, Barnard ND. "Calcium, dairy products, and bone health in children and young adults: a reevaluation of the evidence." Pediatrics. 2005;115:736–743.

40. Feskanich D, Willett WC, Colditz GA. "Calcium, vitamin D, milk consumption, and hip fractures: a prospective study among postmenopausal women." American Journal of Clinical Nutrition. 2003;77:504–511.

41. Bertron P, Barnard ND, Mills M. Racial bias in federal nutrition policy, part I: the public health implications of variations in lactase persistence. Journal of National Medical Association. 1999;91:151–157.

WALKING CHALLENGE

42. "Facts about Physical Activity." Centers for Disease Control and Prevention. Centers for Disease Control and Prevention, 23 May 2014. Web. 12 July 2016. <http://www.cdc.gov/physicalactivity/data/facts.htm>.

43. Nicolaas P. Pronk, PhD; Abigail S. Katz, PhD; Marcia Lowry, MS; Jane Rodmyre Payfer. Reducing "Occupational Sitting Time and Improving Worker Health: The Take-a-Stand Project," 2011, Centers for Disease Control and Prevention

44. "Why Walking?" American Heart Association, 23 June 2014. Web. 8 June 2015. http://www.heart.org/HEARTORG/HealthyLiving/PhysicalActivity/Walking/Why-Walking_UCM_461770_Article.jsp#.V4WiursrLcs

BIBLIOGRAPHY

Babyak, Michael, James A. Blumenthal, Steve Herman, Parinda Khatri, Murali Doraiswamy, Kathleen Moore, W. Edward Craighead, Teri T. Baldewicz, and K. Ranga Krishnan. "Exercise Treatment for Major Depression: Maintenance of Therapeutic Benefit at 10 Months." Psychosomatic Medicine 62.5 (2000): 633-38.

Bermudez, Odilia I., and Xiang Gao. "Greater Consumption of Sweetened Beverages and Added Sugars Is Associated with Obesity among US Young Adults." Annals of Nutrition and Metabolism Ann Nutr Metab 57.3-4 (2010): 211-218.

Charatan, F. "Fluid Intake Affects the Risk of Bladder Cancer in Men." Bmj318.7195 (1999): 1372.

Ciacci, C., C. D'agate, A. De Rosa, C. Franzese, S. Errichiello, V. Gasperi, A. Pardi, D. Quagliata, S. Visentini, and L. Greco. "Self-Rated Quality of Life in Celiac Disease." Digestive Diseases and Sciences 48.11 (2003): 2216-220.

Cordain, Loren, S. Boyd Eaton, Anthony Sebastian, Neil Mann, Staffan Lindeberg, Bruce A. Watkins, James H. O'Keefe, and Janette Brand-Miller. "Origins and Evolution of the Western Diet: Health Implications for the 21st Century1,2." The American Journal of Clinical Nutrition. The American Journal of Clinical Nutrition, Feb. 2005. Web. 12 July 2016. <http://ajcn.nutrition.org/content/81/2/341.full>.

Daussin, F.N., Zoll, J., Dufour, S.P., Ponsot, E., Lonsdorfer-Wolf, E. et al. (2008). Effect of interval versus continuous training on cardiorespiratory and mitochondrial functions; relationship to aerobic performance improvements in sedentary subjects, American Journal of Physiology: Regulatory, Integrative and Comparative Physiology, 295, R264-R272.

Emmons, Robert A., and Cheryl A. Crumpler. "Gratitude as a Human Strength: Appraising the Evidence." Journal of Social and Clinical Psychology 19.1 (2000): 56-69.

Gibala, Martin J., and Sean L. Mcgee. "Metabolic Adaptations to Short-term High-Intensity Interval Training." Exercise and Sports Sciences Reviews 36.2 (2008): 58-63

ibala, Martin J., "Molecular responses to high-intensity interval exercise." Applied Physiology, Nutrition, and Metabolism, 34(3), (2009)428-432.

Helgerud, Jan, Kjetill Hydal, Eivind Wang, Trine Karlsen, Plr Berg, Marius Bjerkaas, Thomas Simonsen, Cecilies Helgesen, Ninal Hjorth, Ragnhild Bach, and Jan Hoff. "Aerobic High-Intensity Intervals Improve VO2max More Than Moderate Training." Medicine & Science in Sports & Exercise39.4 (2007): 665-671.

Hillman, Charles H., Kirk I. Erickson, and Arthur F. Kramer. "Be Smart, Exercise Your Heart: Exercise Effects on Brain and Cognition." Nature Reviews Neuroscience Nat Rev Neuroscience 9.1 (2008): 58-65.

Hurrell, R. F. "Enhanced Iron Absorption from Cereal and Legume Grains by Phytic Acid Degradation." Bioactive Compounds in Foods. ACS Symposium Series 816 (2002): 117-29.

H Perry, C.G.R, Heigenhauser, G.J.F, Bonen, A., and Spriet, L.L. "High-intensity aerobic interval training increases fat and carbohydrate metabolic capacities in human skeletal muscle." Applied Physiology, Nutrition, and Metabolism, (2008). 33(6), 1112-1123.

Laursen, Paul B., and David G. Jenkins. "the Scientific Basis for High-Intensity Interval Training." Sports Medicine 32.1 (2002): 53-73.

Lasocki, Sigismond. "The True Obesity Paradox." Critical Care Medicine 43.1 (2015): 240-241.

Morabia, Alfredo, and Michael C. Costanza. "Does Walking 15 Minutes per Day Keep the Obesity Epidemic Away? Simulation of the Efficacy of a Populationwide Campaign." American Journal of Public Health. American Journal of Public Health 94.3 (2004): 437-440.

Musa, D.I., Adeniran, S.A., Dikko, A.U., and Sayers, S.P. (2009). "The effect of a high-intensity interval training program on high-density lipoprotein cholesterol in young men." Journal of Strength and Conditioning Research, 23(2), 587-592.

Nachbar, MS, and Oppenheim, JD. "Lectins in the United States Diet: A Survey of Lectins in Commonly Consumed Foods and a Review of the Literature." Lectins in the United States Diet: A Survey of Lectins in Commonly Consumed Foods and a 33.11 (1980): 2338-2345.

Ng, Shu Wen, Meghan M. Slining, and Barry M. Popkin. "Use of Caloric and Noncaloric Sweeteners in US Consumer Packaged Foods, 2005-2009."Journal of the Academy of Nutrition and Dietetics 112.11 (2012) 1821-1834.

Novak, W.k, and A.g Haslberger. "Substantial Equivalence of Antinutrients and Inherent Plant Toxins in Genetically Modified Novel Foods." Food and Chemical Toxicology 38.6 (2000): 473-483.

Ogden, Cynthia L., Margaret D. Carroll, Brian K. Kit, and Katherine M. Flegal. "Prevalence of Childhood and Adult Obesity in the United States, 2011–2012." Survey of Anesthesiology 58.4 (2014): 206.

O'keefe, James H., and Loren Cordain. "Cardiovascular Disease Resulting From a Diet and Lifestyle at Odds With Our Paleolithic Genome: How to Become a 21st-Century Hunter-Gatherer." Mayo Clinic Proceedings 79.1 (2004): 101-108.

Owen, Neville, Geneviève N. Healy, Charles E. Matthews, and David W. Dunstan. "Too Much Sitting." Exercise and Sport Sciences Reviews 38.3 (2010): 105-113.

Pellegrina, Chiara Dalla, Omar Perbellini, Maria Teresa Scupoli, Carlo Tomelleri, Chiara Zanetti, Gianni Zoccatelli, Marina Fusi, Angelo Peruffo, Corrado Rizzi, and Roberto Chignola. "Effects of Wheat Germ Agglutinin on Human Gastrointestinal Epithelium: Insights from an Experimental Model of Immune/epithelial Cell Interaction." Toxicology and Applied Pharmacology 237.2 (2009): 146-53.

Pusztai, A., S. W. B. Ewen, G. Grant, D. S. Brown, J. C. Stewart, W. J. Peumans, E. J. M. Van Damme, and S. Bardocz. "Antinutritive Effects of Wheat-germ Agglutinin and Other N-acetylglucosamine-specific Lectins." BJN British Journal of Nutrition 70.01 (1993): 313.

Roberts KM, Noble EG, Hayden DB, Taylor AW. Simple and complex carbohydrate-rich diets and muscle glycogen content of marathon runners. European Journal Applied Physiology. 1988;57(1):70-74.

Sapone, Anna, Karen M. Lammers, Vincenzo Casolaro, Marcella Cammarota, Maria Giuliano, Mario De Rosa, Rosita Stefanile, Giuseppe Mazzarella, Carlo Tolone, Maria Russo, Pasquale Esposito, Franca Ferraraccio, Maria Cartenì, Gabriele Riegler, Laura De Magistris, and Alessio Fasano. "Divergence of Gut Permeability and Mucosal Immune Gene Expression in Two Gluten-associated Conditions: Celiac Disease and Gluten Sensitivity." BMC Medicine 9.1 (2011): 23.

Fat Oxidation during Exercise in Women." Journal of Applied Physiology 102.4 (2006): 1439-1447

Tang, Reiping, Jeng-Yi Wang, Sing-Kai Lo, and Ling-Ling Hsieh. "Physical Activity, Water Intake and Risk of Colorectal Cancer in Taiwan: A Hospital-based Case-control Study." International Journal of Cancer 82.4 (1999): 484-489.

Teismann, T., S. Het, M. Grillenberger, U. Willutzki, and O. T. Wolf. "Writing about Life Goals: Effects on Rumination, Mood and the Cortisol Awakening Response." Journal of Health Psychology 19.11 (2013): 1410-419.

Thompson, Lilian U. "Potential Health Benefits and Problems Associated with Antinutrients in Foods." Food Research International 26.2 (1993): 131-49.

"Types of Carbohydrates." American Diabetes Association. N.p., 9 Mar. 2015. Web. 08 July 2016.

Vasconcelos, Ilka M., and José Tadeu A Oliveira. "Antinutritional Properties of Plant Lectins." Toxicon 44.4 (2004): 385-403.

Via, Michael. "The Malnutrition of Obesity: Micronutrient Deficiencies That Promote Diabetes." ISRN Endocrinology 2012 (2012): 1-8.

Voss, Gretchen. "Sugar Is Killing Us. Here's Everything You Need to Know." Women's Health., 12 June 2014. Web. 8 June 2015. http://www.womenshealthmag.com/health/dangers-of-sugar

Watkins, Philip C. "Introduction: Why a Science of Gratitude?" Gratitude and the Good Life (2013): 1-9.

ACKNOWLEDGEMENTS

The writing of this book has been a labor of love and it couldn't have been completed without the support of friends, family, community members, supportive businesses and my awesome patient participants. You have all inspired me to improve these health challenges and I look forward to serving you in the future. Your support will help improve the lives of countless people. Additionally, I'd like to thank Matt E. for helping to create the catalog of exercises and for organizing the athletes; Jennifer, Lisa, Suzanne, and Emily. Thank you all for being an important part of the First21.

DISCLAIMER

This book is not intended as a substitute for medical advice nor is it intended to diagnose or treat any medical condition. Please consult a licensed healthcare provider before making any healthcare decisions or for guidance about a specific medical condition. Seek professional healthcare advice before beginning any new diet or exercise program. The publisher and author are neither responsible for nor liable for any damages or negative consequences from any action or application to any person reading or following the information in this book.

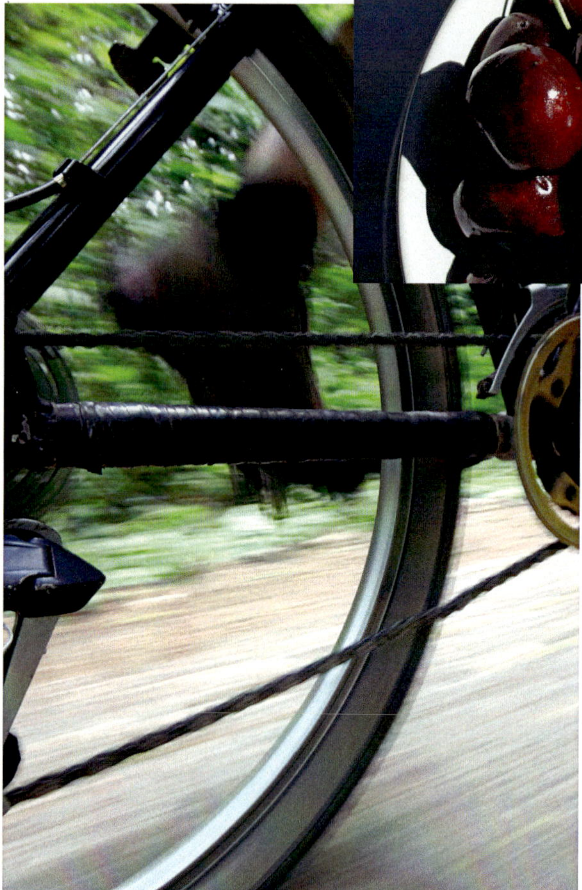

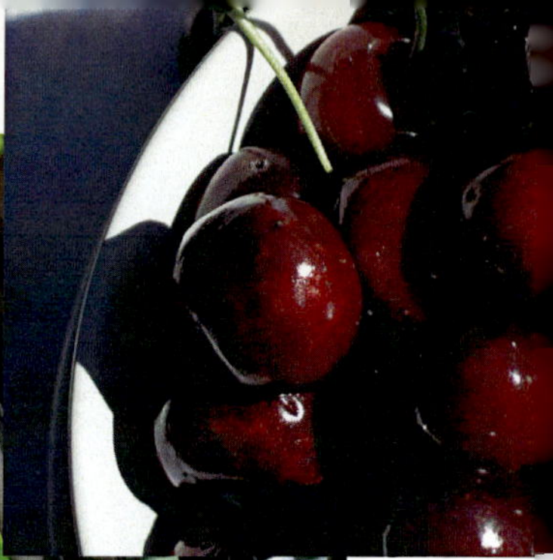

First21.com

First Print 2016 ISBN: 978-0-9978075-0-9